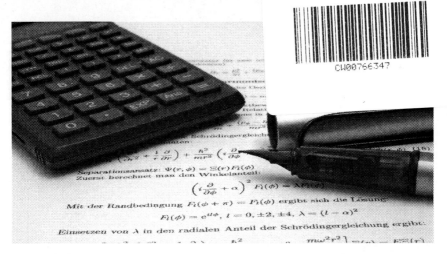

Succeeding in the FRCR Part 1 Exam (Physics Module)

Essential practice MCQs with detailed explanations

Second Edition

Pervinder Bhogal, Thomas Conner, Gauraang Bhatnagar & Harbir Sidhu

Edited by Anmol Malhotra

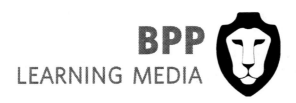

First edition 2009
Second edition November 2011

ISBN 9781 4453 8156 5
Previous ISBN 9781 9068 3918 5
e-ISBN 9781 4453 8577 8

British Library Cataloguing-in-Publication Data
A catalogue record for this book is available from the British Library

Published by
BPP Learning Media Ltd
BPP House, Aldine Place
London W12 8AA

www.bpp.com/health

Typeset by Replika Press Pvt Ltd, India
Printed in the United Kingdom

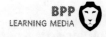

Contents

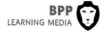

About the Publisher

BPP Learning Media is dedicated to supporting aspiring professionals with top quality learning material. BPP Learning Media's commitment to success is shown by our record of quality, innovation and market leadership in paper-based and e-learning materials. BPP Learning Media's study materials are written by professionally-qualified specialists who know from personal experience the importance of top quality materials for success.

Every effort has been made to ensure the accuracy of the material contained within this guide. However it must be noted that medical treatments, drug dosages/formulations, equipment, procedures and best practice are currently evolving within the field of medicine.

Readers are therefore advised always to check the most up-to-date information relating to:

- The applicable drug manufacturer's product information and data sheets relating to recommended dose/formulation, administration and contraindications.
- The latest applicable local and national guidelines.
- The latest applicable local and national codes of conduct and safety protocols.

It is the responsibility of the practitioner, based on their own knowledge and expertise, to diagnose, treat and ensure the safety and best interests of the patient are maintained.

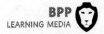

About the Authors

Dr Pervinder Bhogal

Pervinder trained at Royal Free and University College London Medical School and graduated in 2004. After university he passed his MRCS Exam and is currently studying for a Masters Degree in Medical Education. He entered radiology training in 2007 and passed his FRCR Part 1 on the first attempt.

Thomas Conner

Thomas gained a First Class Honours degree in Anatomy and Developmental Biology and graduated in Medicine from University College London in 2004. He is currently a radiology registrar on the Royal Free Hospital radiology rotation. He is interested in academic radiology.

Gauraang Bhatnagar

Gauraang is a radiology registrar on the Peninsula training scheme. He moved to the South West in 2008 after completing basic surgical training in London. A firm believer in the statement "he's a doctor not a physicist" (Dr Leonard 'Bones' McCoy, Star Trek), he found question books such as this one the ideal way to revise for the FRCR Part 1.

Harbir Sidhu

Harbir graduated from University College London Medical School in 2004. After undertaking basic surgical training in the Yorkshire deanery, he moved to the Southwest. He is currently working in the Peninsula training scheme as a radiology registrar.

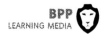

About the Editor

Anmol Malhotra

Anmol completed his radiology training at Barts and the London NHS Trust in February 2005 and spent time as an observer in MRI imaging at Memorial Sloan-Kettering, New York. Anmol now works as a consultant at the Royal Free Hospital in London.

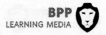

Contributors

Yen Zhi Tang
Radiology registrar, Royal Free radiology rotation

Ynyr Hughes-Roberts
Radiology registrar, Cambridge University Hospital radiology rotation

Dedication

*To our friends and families for
all their love and support*

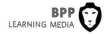

Abbreviations

ARSAC	Administration of Radioactive Substances Advisory Committee
Bq	Becquerel (disintegrations/second)
c	Speed of light (3×10^8 m/s)
C	Coulomb
CTDI	Computed Tomography Dose Index
DAP	Dose Area Product (Gy cm^2)
DRL	Diagnostic Reference Level
eV	Electron volt (1 eV = 1.6×10^{-19} joules)
f	Frequency
FFD	Focus Film Distance
Gy	Gray
H	Planck's constant (6.626×10^{-34} Js)
HVL	Half Value Layer
HSE	Health and Safety Executive
IRR 1999	Ionising Radiations Regulations 1999
IRMER	Ionising Radiation (Medical Exposure) Regulations 2000
kVp	Peak electrical potential across an X-ray tube
LAC	Linear Attenuation Co-efficient
lp/mm	Line pairs per millimeter
mA	Milliamperes
mAs	Milliampere – seconds
MTF	Modulation Transfer Function
SI	Systeme Internationale
Sv	Sievert – the unit of effective dose and equivalent dose
Z	Atomic Number

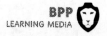

Preface

The FRCR Part 1 Examination for the Fellowship of the Royal College of Radiologists is the first in a series of examinations that radiology registrars must undertake in order to gain membership to the College.

This book is a comprehensive, all-in-one revision guide for candidates. Comprising over a thousand Multiple Choice Questions (MCQs) which test the exact topics on which candidates are examined, the answers to each question are explained in-depth, introducing additional detail so as to cover every subject fully and ensure your success.

We offer you the opportunity to test yourself using questions structured to reflect those in the real examination, and at the same time bring your knowledge up to the required level. Our intention is that by careful revision using this book alongside the standard texts, you will be equipped to pass what is for many a daunting examination.

This book provides up-to-date questions to keep abreast of developments in CT, MRI and Nuclear Medicine, and with sections on MRI and Ultrasound physics we address challenging topics more recently introduced into the examination.

As well as FRCR Part 1 candidates, we believe that this book will be extremely useful for the following readership:

- Radiologists sitting FRCR Part 2b, for which physics knowledge is again required
- Foundation Year doctors interested in applying for radiology
- Radiographers undertaking training
- Outside of the UK, graduates undergoing radiology training.

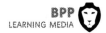

We hope that you will find this book easy-to-use and essential to your preparation.

Good luck in your studies!

Dr Anmol Malhotra
Consultant radiologist
Royal Free Hampstead NHS Trust

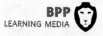

About the exam and tips on passing it

The first FRCR examination expects candidates to understand and demonstrate knowledge of the physical principles that underpin diagnostic medical imaging, and of the anatomy needed to perform and interpret radiological studies. The examination is held three times a year and comprises a physics and a radiological anatomy module. All candidates will need to pass both modules in order to pass the examination but the modules can be sat separately. There is no limit on the number of times a candidate may sit the exam and no time limit to passing it.

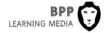

Format of the exam

The physics module comprises 40 MCQ's and the examination lasts for two hours. It is not negatively marked. The pass mark varies for the exam depending upon the difficulty but is usually in the region of 60-70%.

Revision tips

Physics is not everyone's favourite subject but regular study followed by self-assessment is the best way to prepare for this examination. In order to give yourself the best chance at passing the examination at the first attempt, start preparing approximately 2-3 months in advance. This book should help save time nearer to the exam, as the explanations should refresh knowledge gained from other more comprehensive texts and lectures.

Tips for the exam
- Manage your time carefully
- Read the questions and select your answers carefully
- If you are unsure, skip the question and you can go back to it afterwards
- Guess any questions at the end because there is no negative marking, so it is worth putting an answer down
- Check for silly mistakes if you still have time
- Keep watching the clock (40 questions in two hours).

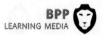

How to use this book

Each of the chapters in this book contains a series of FRCR Part 1 examination topics. Every topic contains five multiple choice statements labelled A-E that are true or false; your task is to determine which.

Below each set of questions is a section of text in which the topic is discussed, and the answers are revealed in context. Then follows a formal statement of the test answers.

For ease of use, we have chosen to show the discussion and answers directly below each set of questions, rather than making you turn to the back of the book for them. This means that to make best use of this book, you should tackle each question honestly, covering the answers and avoiding the temptation to look until you have arrived at your own responses.

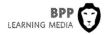

Chapter 1

Basic atomic structure, radioactive decay

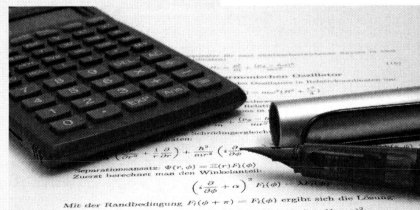

Basic atomic structure, radioactive decay

Please answer all questions true or false. There is no negative marking.

---

1. Concerning the nucleus of atoms
   A. It is made up of protons and electrons
   B. It is made up of protons and neutrons
   C. Nucleons are held together by the strong nuclear force
   D. The mass number represents the number of protons
   E. The number of protons and neutrons is always equal

The nucleus of an atom is composed of protons and neutrons. The charge of protons is +1 and it is 0 for neutrons. The strong nuclear force is responsible for holding the nucleus together. The mass number represents the number of protons and neutrons, whereas it is the atomic number that represents the number of protons only. The number of protons and neutrons is not always equal, and for higher atomic number elements neutrons tend to outnumber protons.

---

1. A. **False** – it is made of protons and neutrons
   B. **True** – it is made of protons and neutrons
   C. **True** – the strong nuclear force holds nucleons (protons and neutrons) together
   D. **False** – the mass number is the number of protons and neutrons
   E. **False** – the number of protons and neutrons is not always equal

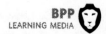

2. Concerning electrons
   A. In the Bohr model of atomic structure electrons orbit the nucleus
   B. The electron has +1 charge
   C. The binding energy of the L-shell is higher than the K-shell
   D. The K-shell can hold 2 electrons
   E. Electrons have a greater mass than protons

In the Bohr model of the nucleus electrons orbit the nucleus in discrete energy shells. These energy shells start with the letter K and increase alphabetically, eg K,L,M,N,O, etc. Each shell holds a certain number of electrons. The energy required to remove an electron from its shell is referred to as the electron binding energy. This is greatest for the inner shell electrons (K-shell) and decreases the further away the electron is from the nucleus. Electrons have a smaller mass than protons, at approximately 9.1×10^{-31} Kg. The mass of a proton is approximately 1836 times greater than this.

---

2. A. **True** – in the Bohr model electrons orbit the nucleus
   B. **False** – the electron has a charge of -1
   C. **False** – the binding energy for the K-shell is higher than for the L-shell
   D. **True** – the K-shell can hold 2 electrons
   E. **False** – protons have much greater mass than electrons

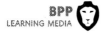

---

3. Concerning the atomic number of tungsten
   A. It has an atomic number of 74
   B. It has a physical density of approximately 19
   C. The K-shell binding energy of tungsten is 20
   D. The mass number of tungsten is 284
   E. It is represented by the letter W

Tungsten is an important element in radiology as it is used to produce X-rays. It is represented by the letter W. It has an atomic number of 74 and mass number 184 (110 neutrons). The K-shell binding energy of tungsten is 69.5 KeV. Molybdenum has a K-Shell binding energy of 20.0 KeV.

---

3. A. **True** – atomic number is 74
   B. **True** – tungsten has a physical density of approximately 19
   C. **False** – the K-shell binding energy for tungsten is 69.5 KeV
   D. **False** – the mass number for tungsten is 184
   E. **True** – it is represented by the letter W on the periodic table

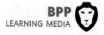

4. Concerning the isotopes of an element
   A. They have the same number of neutrons
   B. They have the same physical properties
   C. They have the same chemical properties
   D. All isotopes are stable
   E. I^{123} decays by emitting gamma rays

Isotopes of an element have the same number of protons and different numbers of neutrons. They have similar chemical properties and different physical properties. Not all isotopes are stable and hence they can be used in imaging using radio-nuclides. Iodine 123 decays by emitting 160 KeV gamma rays and it is used in the imaging of the thyroid gland.

4. A. **False** – isotopes have different numbers of neutrons
   B. **False** – they have different physical properties
   C. **True** – they have the same chemical properties
   D. **False** – not all isotopes are stable
   E. **True** – I^{123} decays by gamma emission

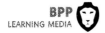

5. Concerning nuclides
   A. Unstable nuclides are called radionuclides
   B. Nuclides with the same number of protons are called isotopes
   C. Nuclides with the same number of neutrons are called isobars
   D. Isobars have the same atomic mass numbers
   E. An isomer is a nucleus in an unexcited state

Isotopes have the same number of protons. Isotones have the same number of neutrons. Isobars have the same atomic mass numbers. An isomer is the excited state of a nucleus.

---

5. A. **True** – unstable nuclides are termed radionuclides
   B. **True** – isotopes have the same number of protons but a different number of neutrons
   C. **False** – nuclides with the same number of neutrons are called isotones
   D. **True** – isobars have the same atomic mass number
   E. **False** – an isomer is a nucleus in an excited state

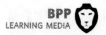

6. Regarding radioactive half-life
   A. It is constant for a particular radionuclide
   B. Decay is a stochastic event
   C. Half-life is defined as the time taken for half the material to decay
   D. Half-life is directly proportional to the decay constant
   E. One Curie is one transformation per second

Radioactive half-life is the time taken for half the material to decay. The decay constant is equal to 0.693/half-life. The activity is the number of transformations in unit time. The Becquerel is 1 transformation per second. The Curie is 3.7×10^{10} transformations per second. Radioactive decay is an exponential process and as such the activity will **never** become 0.

---

6. A. **True** – for a particular radionuclide the half-life is constant
   B. **True** – radioactive decay is a stochastic event
   C. **True** – this is the definition
   D. **False** – it is inversely proportional to the half-life
   E. **False** – a Becquerel is one transformation per second

Definition STOCHASTIC – random probability distribution or pattern that can be statistically analysed but not precisely predicted

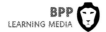

7. Concerning alpha decay
   A. It occurs only in light nuclei
   B. It results in the atomic number decreasing by 4
   C. The alpha particle is equal to the hydrogen nucleus
   D. Alpha particles have an energy between 4-7 MeV
   E. It does not occur in nature

The alpha particle consists of 2 neutrons and 2 protons. It is the equivalent of a helium nucleus. It generally occurs with heavy atoms with atomic numbers greater than 82. Alpha particles have a high energy and as such are very damaging to living tissues. They carry a charge of +2 and can travel up to 10 cm in air. In tissues they travel less than 0.1 mm. They have an energy between 4-7 MeV. They cause the atomic number to fall by 2 and the atomic mass number to fall by 4.

---

7. A. **False** – it occurs in heavy nuclei
   B. **False** – the atomic number decreases by 2
   C. **False** – the alpha particle is the equivalent to a helium nucleus
   D. **True** – they do have an energy between 4-7 MeV
   E. **False** – alpha decay does occur in nature

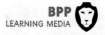

8. Concerning beta plus decay
   A. It is also called positron emission
   B. It occurs in nuclei that are neutron rich
   C. The atomic number decreases by 1
   D. A neutron is emitted with the positron
   E. A positron has a charge of −1

Beta plus decay is also called positron emission decay. A positron is an electron with a +1 charge and is a form of anti-matter. It occurs in nuclei which are neutron poor. A proton is converted to a neutron and positron which is ejected from the atom. In addition to the positron a neutrino (not a neutron) is ejected.

---

8. A. **True** – beta plus decay is also called positron emission
   B. **False** – it occurs in neutron poor nuclei
   C. **True** – the atomic number decreases by 1
   D. **False** – the neutron is not emitted
   E. **False** – a positron has a charge of +1

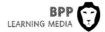

9.   Regarding positrons
   A.   Positrons have a mass equal to electrons
   B.   They annihilate with electrons and release one 511 KeV photon
   C.   Fluorine[18] (F^{18}) is a positron emitter
   D.   Elements that decay by positron emission have long half-lives
   E.   Positrons only exist while they have kinetic energy

Positrons only exist while they have kinetic energy. When they come to rest they spontaneously annihilate with an electron. The mass of the positron and the electron is converted into two photons with energy of 511 KeV that are emitted in exact opposite directions (180 degrees apart.)

Some important positron emitters are F^{18}, O^{15} and C^{11}. Positron emitters generally have short $T_{1/2}$.

9.   A.   **True** – positrons and electrons have the same mass but opposite charge
   B.   **False** – two photons are released
   C.   **True** – F^{18} is a positron emitter
   D.   **False** – they tend to have short half-lives
   E.   **True** – positrons only exist while they have kinetic energy

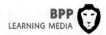

10. Concerning beta minus decay
    A. Phosphorus^{32} (P^{32}) is a pure beta minus emitter
    B. Beta minus decay occurs in neutron-rich radionuclides
    C. The electrons are emitted from the orbital shells
    D. The atomic number increases by 1
    E. An anti-neutrino is emitted alongside the electron

In beta minus decay, a neutron in the nucleus is converted to a proton. An electron and an anti-neutrino are ejected in the process. This process occurs in neutron-rich nuclei. The electrons released have a wide range of energies up to a maximum dependent on the emmiting nuclide. The mass number remains the same, but the atomic number will increase by 1.

10. A. **True** – P^{32} is a pure beta minus emitter
    B. **True** – it occurs in neutron rich radionuclides
    C. **False** – the electrons are ejected from the nucleus
    D. **True** – the atomic number increases by 1
    E. **True** – an anti-neutrino is ejected alongside the electron

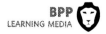

11. The following are part of the Electromagnetic (EM) spectrum
    A. Sound waves
    B. Microwaves
    C. Ultraviolet light
    D. Alpha particles
    E. X-rays

The electromagnetic spectrum is a continuum stretching from radio waves to gamma and X-rays. Electromagnetic radiation travels in straight lines at the speed of light – c (3×10^8 m/sec in a vacuum). An electromagnetic wave is made up of two waves, a electric wave and magnetic wave that oscillate perpendicular to their direction of motion and at 90 degrees to each other. These are examples of transverse waves.

---

11. A. **False** – not part of EM spectrum
    B. **True** – part of the EM spectrum
    C. **True** – part of the EM spectrum
    D. **False** – represents 2 neutrons and 2 protons
    E. **True** – part of the EM spectrum

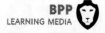

12. Concerning electromagnetic radiation
  A. It travels at a constant speed independent of the matter through which it travels
  B. Wavelength and frequency are directly related
  C. The product of wavelength and frequency is constant
  D. Electromagnetic radiation exists as photons
  E. X-rays and gamma rays always have different frequency and wavelength

---

Electromagnetic radiation exists in discrete packages of energy called photons. These photons can behave as waves and particles, so-called 'wave particle duality.' The energy of a photon is related to the wavelength and frequency.

Photon energy: $E = h \times f$ where f = frequency and h is Planck's constant.

Since $f = 1/$wavelength, the energy is directly related to the frequency and inversely related to wavelength.

Electromagnetic radiation does travel at a constant speed, but this speed is related to the medium through which it travels. The product of wavelength and frequency is equal to the speed of light, c.

X-rays and gamma rays cannot be distinguished in terms of frequency and wavelength. They are called X-rays if they are produced by electron interactions and gamma rays if they are produced by nuclear reactions.

---

12. A. **False** – the speed is dependant on the matter
  B. **False** – wavelength and frequency are indirectly related
  C. **True** – constant is 1
  D. **True** – electromagnetic radiation exists as photons
  E. **False** – they cannot be distinguished by frequency and wavelength

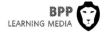

13.   Regarding electron capture
   A.   It occurs in radionuclides with a neutron deficit
   B.   It is most likely with valence electrons
   C.   A neutron combines with the electron to produce a
        proton
   D.   The atomic number decreases by 1
   E. I^{123} decays wholly by electron capture

In this form of decay a proton captures an electron from one of the shells and is converted into a neutron. It occurs in nuclei that are neutron poor. The electron is most likely to be absorbed from the K-shell then from the L, M, N, etc. The loss of the electron from the shell leaves a hole which needs to be filled. This hole can be filled by an electron from another shell. This process can cause the emission of K characteristic X-rays. I^{123} decays by electron capture and produces 160 KeV gamma rays and 28 KeV X-rays.

13.   A.   **True** – it occurs in neutron poor radionuclides
      B.   **False** – it is most likely to occur with K-shell electrons
      C.   **False** – an electron combines with a proton to form a
                neutron
      D.   **True** – since a proton is converted into a neutron
      E.   **True** – after electron capture gamma and X-rays are
                produced

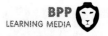

14. The following are correctly paired
    A. Alpha decay decreases the mass number by 4
    B. Beta minus decay increases the atomic number by 1
    C. Electron capture increases the atomic number by 1
    D. Beta plus decay increases the number of neutrons by 1
    E. Alpha decay decreases the atomic number by 2

There are several decay modes. In alpha decay the radionuclide emits an alpha particle that consists of 2 neutrons and 2 protons (a helium nucleus). This is most common in atoms with atomic numbers above 82. The loss of 2 neutrons and 2 protons causes the mass number to decrease by 4 and the atomic number to decrease by 2.

In beta minus decay, a neutron inside the nucleus is converted into a proton, and the excess energy is released in the form of a beta particle and an antineutrino. Beta minus decay occurs in nuclei that are neutron rich. Hence, in beta minus decay the atomic number increases by 1 but the mass number remains the same.

In beta plus decay (also known as positron emission) a proton inside the nucleus is converted into a neutron and the excess energy is emitted as a positron (a positively charged electron) and a neutrino. Beta plus decay tends to occur in nuclei with too few neutrons. In beta plus decay, the atomic number decreases by 1 and the mass number remains the same.

Electron capture occurs when a proton inside the nucleus is converted into a neutron by capturing an electron from one of its atomic shells. A neutrino is emitted in the process. It occurs in nuclei with too few neutrons and may compete with beta plus decay. If the electron is captured from the K-shell, an outer shell electron fills the vacancy left in the K-shell. The excess energy is emitted as either an Auger electron or characteristic X-rays. Electron capture results in a decrease in the atomic number by 1 and an increase in the mass number by 1.

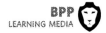

14. A. **True** – the mass number decreases by 4 in alpha decay
    B. **True** – beta minus decay increases the atomic number by 1
    C. **False** – electron capture decreases the atomic number by 1
    D. **True** – beta plus decay increases the number of neutrons by 1
    E. **True** – alpha decay decreases the atomic number by 2

15. The linear energy transfer (LET)
   A. LET represents the energy deposited in tissue per unit length
   B. High LET radiations are easily stopped
   C. Gamma rays have lower LET than neutrons
   D. Alpha particles have the highest LET
   E. High LET radiation damage is more likely to be non-repairable

The linear energy transfer is a way of expressing the energy deposited in a medium per unit path length. Larger particles and more heavily charged particles are more easily stopped. These large charged particles have a higher LET since they deposit their energy in a shorter length. Alpha particles have the highest LET followed by neutrons, beta particles and X-rays, and gamma rays have the lowest LET.

15. A. **True** – this is a basic definition for the linear energy transfer
   B. **True** – larger, more highly charged particles are more easily stopped
   C. **True** – gamma rays have a lower LET than neutrons
   D. **True** – alpha particles are the heaviest and highest charged therefore have the highest LET
   E. **True** – the damage is more severe because of the higher energy deposited

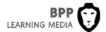

16. Radioactive material
    A. Does not occur in nature
    B. Is important in radiology
    C. Decays to produce sound waves
    D. Decays to a level of 0
    E. Decays by a factor of approx. 250 times after 8 half-lives

Radioactive material does occur in nature from many sources. Sound waves are not produced in the decay process, but electromagnetic radiation may be produced. Radioactive material will never reach a level of 0 because the decay is exponential. After 8 half-lives the level of radioactivity will be 256 times lower than the initial level.

16. A. **False** – radioactive material is found in nature
    B. **True** – it forms the basis of nuclear imaging
    C. **False** – it does not decay to produce sound waves
    D. **False** – it never reaches 0 but becomes asymptotic with 0
    E. **True** – 2^8 is 256

17. The following are positron emitters
    A. Carbon 11
    B. Indium 111
    C. Nitrogen 13
    D. Oxygen 15
    E. Fluorine 18

Positron emitters are not widely used in medical radiology. They are cyclotron-produced. A cyclotron bombards nuclei with high energy protons to create unstable nuclei that are proton rich. These will then tend to decay by positron emission (beta plus emission).

17. A. **True** – emits positrons
    B. **False** – emits gamma rays
    C. **True** – emits positrons
    D. **True** – emits positrons
    E. **True** – emits positrons

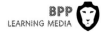

18. Metastable states
    A. Are stable
    B. Must have a $T_{1/2}$ longer than 10^{-12} seconds
    C. Can be generator-produced
    D. Can decay by isomeric transition
    E. Both the parent and daughter nuclides may have the same atomic number and mass number after decay

---

Metastable states are unstable. They are represented by a lower case 'm' after the mass number. By definition a metastable state must have a half-life over longer than 10^{-12} seconds. They can be generator-produced, and technetium 99 m is an important generator-produced radionuclide used in medical radiology. After decay by isomeric transition the mass number, atomic number and neutron number all remain unchanged.

---

18. A. **False** – they are unstable
    B. **True** – this is part of the definition
    C. **True** – they can be produced in a generator
    D. **True** – they can decay by isomeric transition
    E. **True** – after isomeric decay atomic number, mass number and neutron number are unchanged

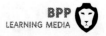

19. I^{123} and I^{125} have different
A. Chemical properties
B. Physical properties
C. Numbers of neutrons
D. Numbers of protons
E. Numbers of valence electrons if uncharged

Isomers have different physical properties and the same chemical properties. They have different numbers of neutrons and the same number of protons. Change in the number of valence electrons will cause the atoms to become ions not isomers.

---

19. A. **False** – isotopes have the same chemical properties
B. **True** – isotopes have different physical properties
C. **True** – isotopes have different number of neutrons
D. **False** – isotopes have the same number of protons
E. **False** – isotopes will have the same number of valence electrons if uncharged

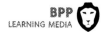

20. Regarding the inverse square law
    A. The intensity will be 1/8 if the distance doubles
    B. It applies to all electromagnetic radiation
    C. It represents energy conservation principles
    D. Applies to all sources of radiation
    E. Can be used in protection radiation

The inverse square law is an important principle in physics. For a point source it states that the intensity will be proportional to the square of the distance from the point source. So if the distance doubles the intensity will decrease by 4 times, etc. The law applies to all radiation from the electromagnetic spectrum as long as it is a point source. It does represent a conservation of energy principle. The inverse square law is useful in radiation protection, as the radiologist can relatively easily increase the distance between themselves and the radiation source and hence cut the intensity they are exposed to.

20. A. **False** – the intensity will 1/4
     B. **True** – the inverse square law applies to all electro-magnetic radiation
     C. **True** – it represents energy conservation
     D. **False** – it applies to all radiation from a point source
     E. **True** – it is very important in radiation protection

Chapter 2
Production of X-rays

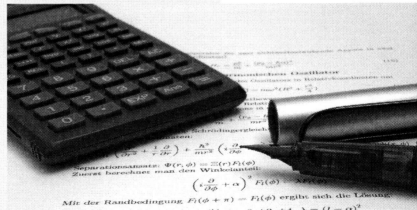

Production of X-rays

Please answer all questions true or false. There is no negative marking.

1. The cathode of the X-ray tube
    A. Is commonly made of tungsten
    B. Has a high melting point
    C. Has a low resistance
    D. Is positively charged in relation to the anode
    E. Can exceed temperatures of 2200°C

The cathode of a typical X-ray tube is commonly made of a coiled wire of tungsten. This metal is chosen because it has a high melting point and low vapour pressure (few electrons are evaporated off the surface). The process of producing electrons is called thermionic emission. Tungsten has a relatively high resistance and this is needed to reach the high temperatures required to achieve thermionic emission. The temperature can exceed 2200°C. The cathode is negatively charged in relation to the anode.

---

1. A. **True** – the cathode is commonly made from a coiled wire of tungsten
    B. **True** – it must have a high melting point
    C. **False** – the resistance needs to be high
    D. **False** – the cathode is negatively charged
    E. **True** – the temperature can exceed 2200°C

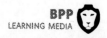

2. Concerning the anode
    A. It is positively charged relative to the cathode
    B. Molybdenum is used in most X-ray tubes
    C. Rhodium is often added to tungsten to reduce pitting and cracking that can be caused by overheating
    D. The distance between the cathode and anode affects the quality of the X-rays produced
    E. 90% of the energy from the electrons striking the anode is dissipated as heat

---

The anode in most X-ray tubes is composed of a tungsten/rhenium alloy. The rhenium is added to prevent pitting and cracking of the anode caused by the high temperatures, which would decrease the life expectancy of the tube, the efficiency of X-ray production and the quality of the beam. Molybdenum is used in mammography tubes. The distance between the anode and cathode has no effect on the quality of the beam. 99% of the energy is dissipated as heat and only 1% is converted to X-rays.

---

2. A. **True** – the anode is positively charged in relation to the cathode
    B. **False** – the anode is a tungsten/rhenium alloy in most tubes
    C. **False** – rhenium is added
    D. **False** – this has no effect
    E. **False** – 99% is dissipated as heat

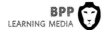

> 3.   The X-ray tube
>   A.   Envelope is housed in oil to help lubricate the motor bearings
>   B.   Envelope contains a vacuum
>   C.   Housing does not contain shielding to prevent radiation leakage
>   D.   Envelope is generally constructed from thick lead
>   E.   Housing oil can be used as a temperature sensitive switch

The X-ray tube envelope is commonly made of thick walled glass. In it are the cathode, anode and vacuum. Metal envelopes are also available. The vacuum is needed to prevent the electrons produced at the cathode from striking gas molecules as they travel towards the anode. This would significantly impede the efficiency of the X-ray tube. The housing has several functions that include the following:

•   Lead-lined and so shields against leakage/stray radiation
•   Allows the mounting of the envelope and the tube itself
•   Electrical insulation by means of oil
•   Provides electrical contact terminals
•   Contains a window through which the X-rays pass after being produced. Some attenuation occurs at this point.

The oil that is found in the housing serves several purposes:

•   Electrical insulation
•   Dissipation of heat via convection
•   It can be used as a switch. As the heat is absorbed by the oil it will expand. This expansion will continue with further heating. A switch – Expansion Diaphragm – can be triggered when the oil has expanded a certain amount and so can prevent over-heating of the system.

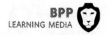

3.   A.   **False** – the oil is not used to lubricate the bearings
     B.   **True** – this is needed to prevent the electrons from striking gas molecules
     C.   **False** – contains a lead lining to act as shielding
     D.   **False** – the envelope is commonly thick walled glass
     E.   **True** – the housing oil can be used as a temperature dependant switch

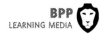

4.   Regarding the X-ray tube filament
      A.   Typically, it has a current of 4A
      B.   It has a typical power dissipation of 40W
      C.   There is a surrounding space charge of positive charge
            that repels the electrons away from the cathode and
            towards the anode
      D.   Tube filament current and tube current are the
            same
      E.   It is surrounded by a focusing cup

The cathode filament is typically made of tungsten, with a current of 4A and voltage of 10V. It therefore has a typical power dissipation of 40W. Two filaments may be found within the same X-ray tube and these can be used to produce different-sized focal spots. The filament has a focusing cup which acts like a lens to target the electrons onto a small spot on the anode. If two filaments are present then two focusing cups are needed. The tube filament current and the tube current are **not** the same. The filament current is that present across the filament itself. The tube current is the current flowing from anode to cathode.

Surrounding the filament is the space charge. This is a cloud of negatively charged electrons that act to prevent the further emission of electrons. As a result of this space charge, below a certain tube voltage electrons will not travel from the cathode to the anode and so no X-rays will be produced – a 'space charge limited' operation. Hence a certain minimum operating voltage is required.

4.   A.   **True** – this is a typical current
      B.   **True** – this is the typical power dissipation
      C.   **False** – the space charge is with negatively charged
                  electrons
      D.   **False** – these are not the same. Tube filament current is
                  the current across the filament, and tube current
                  is the current between anode and cathode
      E.   **True** – the focusing cup acts as a lens to target the
                  electrons

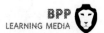

5.   Rotating anodes
      A.   Use induction motors
      B.   Are mounted on rods with a high conductivity
      C.   Use oil-lubricated bearings to minimise heat
           conduction
      D.   Have an anode diameter of approximately 10 cm
      E.   Increase the area over which heat is dissipated

Rotating anodes are now commonly used in X-ray tubes. They allow a much larger area to be bombarded by electrons because the disc is rotating. This increase in the area of bombardment also increases the area of heat loss, that in turn results in an increase in the tube rating. To maintain the vacuum in the envelope the motors use electrical induction to rotate. Silver, never oil, is often used as the lubricant for the bearings. To prevent the bearings from overheating and hence seizing up, the anode stem must be made of a low-conductivity metal such as molybdenum.

5.   A.   **True** – induction motors are used in rotating anodes
      B.   **False** – they are mounted on low conductivity rods
      C.   **False** – oil is not used to lubricate the bearings
      D.   **True** – this is a common size for a rotating anode
      E.   **True** – rotating the anode increases the area over which
                     electrons strike it and hence generates heat

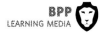

6.   The following focal spot size and clinical application are
      correctly paired
      A.   0.01 to 0.015 mm for magnification mammography
      B.   0.1–0.15 mm for magnification mammography
      C.   0.6 mm for fluoroscopy
      D.   0.3 mm for magnification radiography
      E.   1.2 mm for conventional radiography with small
            focal spot

The following focal spot sizes and applications are found:

*   0.1–0.15 mm   magnification mammography
*   0.3 mm   mammography and magnification radiology
*   0.6 mm   conventional radiography (small focal spot)
                   and fluoroscopy
*   1.2 mm   conventional radiography (large focal spot)

6.   A.   **False** – 0.1–0.15 mm
      B.   **True** – 0.1–0.15 mm
      C.   **True** – 0.6 mm
      D.   **True** – 0.3 mm
      E.   **False** – 0.6 mm

7.   Concerning the actual focal spot
     A.   It is the area on the anode over which heat is produced
     B.   Increasing the target angle will decrease the actual focal spot
     C.   Increasing mA decreases the effectiveness of focusing
     D.   It can be measured using a pinhole camera technique
     E.   Increasing the actual focal spot decreases the tube loading

---

The actual focal spot is the area on the anode over which heat is produced. It determines the tube rating. Since a larger actual focal spot can dissipate heat over a larger area the tube rating will be higher. However, this will alter the effective focal spot and hence unsharpness etc. Increasing the target angle will increase the actual focal spot size. Increasing the mA will decrease the effectiveness of focusing. This is called blooming, and it is caused by the electrostatic repulsion of the electrons. This effect will cause an increase in the focal spot size. Focal spot sizes can be measured using pinhole cameras, star or bar test patterns and slit cameras.

---

7.   A.   **True** – this is the definition
     B.   **False** – increasing the target angle increases the actual focal spot size
     C.   **True** – this is called blooming
     D.   **True** – this is one way to test the actual focal spot size
     E.   **False** – increasing the focal spot size increases the tube loading

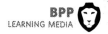

8. Concerning the target angle
    A. It is generally between 7^0 and 20^0
    B. It is the angle between the target surface and the central beam
    C. Steeper angles result in larger fields of coverage
    D. Mammography uses a steep target angle
    E. Smaller target angles improve fine detail imaging

The target angle is the angle between the target surface and the central beam. It is usually between 7° and 20°. A steeper target angle (smaller angle) results in a narrower effective focal spot. This means a smaller field of coverage but improvement in the geometrical unsharpness. Mammography requires fine detail imaging and only needs a narrow field of view; therefore it is suited to steeper target angles.

---

8. A. **True** – it is normally between 7° and 20°
    B. **True** – this is how the target angle is measured
    C. **False** – a steeper angle means a narrower effective focal spot and smaller field of coverage
    D. **True** – mammography does use a steep target angle
    E. **True** – by improving geometrical unsharpness

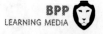

9.   In diagnostic X-ray tubes
      A.   The rotating anode may rotate at up to 10000 rpm
      B.   Convection currents are set up in the housing oil
      C.   Conduction is the primary method of heat
           dissipation
      D.   10% of the electrical energy used is converted to
           X-rays
      E.   An ionisation chamber is fitted between the anode
           and cathode

In modern X-ray tubes with rotating anodes the anode may rotate at between 3000 and 10000 rpm. This allows the heat produced at the target to be spread over a larger area. Heat generated at the target surface must be dissipated. The three ways that heat can be dissipated are radiation, convection and conduction. All three methods are used within the X-ray tube. Heat radiation to the insulating oil is the main method for heat dissipation. This is aided by blackening the anode surface. This loss of heat by radiation increases as the temperature of the anode increases. Heat loss is proportional to Temp ^{4} (Kelvin). This heat is then transferred by convection to the tube housing. Conduction also occurs within the anode. Some of this heat is conducted along the anode stem. This must be kept to a minimum to prevent the rotors from seizing, hence poorly conducting materials are chosen for the stem. Ionisation chambers are not fitted between the anode and cathode. Only 1% of the energy is converted to X-rays.

9.   A.   **True** – it may rotate between 3000–10000 rpm
      B.   **True** – convection currents flow in the oil
      C.   **False** – radiation is the main method for heat
                dissipation
      D.   **False** – 1% of the electrical energy used is converted
                into X-rays
      E.   **False** – there is a vacuum between the anode and
                cathode

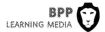

10. With regard to voltage waveform rectification
    A. It converts DC to AC
    B. It uses capacitors in parallel for rectification of the current
    C. Rectification has no effect on X-ray beam quality
    D. Full wave rectification requires a minimum of 4 diodes
    E. Unrectified current can produce X-rays

The current from the national grid is alternating current (AC) – it flows both ways. Rectification is the process by which AC is converted to direct current (DC), in which the current flows one way. This is achieved by using diodes. At least 4 diodes are needed to achieve full wave rectification. Whilst unrectified current can produce X-rays, it is highly inefficient. Rectification will affect the quality of the beam.

10. A. **False** – it converts AC to DC
    B. **False** – it uses diodes not capacitors
    C. **False** – rectification affects the beam quality
    D. **True** – full wave rectification needs at least 4 diodes
    E. **True** – unrectified current can produce X-rays

11. Regarding the X-ray beam quality
     A. X-ray beams are monochromatic
     B. Quality is unaffected by the tube kVp
     C. Increasing peak kVp increases mean beam energy
     D. Decreasing voltage waveform ripple improves beam quality
     E. Filtration has no effect on beam quality

X-ray beam quality relates to the effective photon energy of the X-rays. The effective X-ray energy is an average of the photon energies of a typical polychromatic X-ray beam, and it is typically one third to one half of the maximum photon energy. Things that will affect the quality of the beam are those that will affect the mean energy. Hence:

- Increasing kVp increases the beam quality.
- Reducing voltage waveform ripple will increase the average energy of the X-ray photons. This will increase beam quality. For a three-phase 12-pulse system the ripple is approximately 4%. For a three-phase 6-pulse system the ripple is approximately 14%. So the 12-pulse system will have increased beam quality.
- Appropriate tube filtration should selectively remove low energy photons from the beam as these generally contribute little to the image and increase patient dose. Removing the lower energy photons will increase the mean energy of the beam and hence increase the quality. This is known as beam hardening.

Increasing the beam quality will increase the penetrating power of the beam. This equates to an increase in the half-value layer (HVL) of a material. Increasing the beam quality will also reduce patient dose since fewer lower energy bremsstrahlung X-rays are produced, which contribute more to patient absorbed dose than they do to image formation.

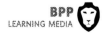

11. A. **False** – X-ray beams are polychromatic
    B. **False** – increasing the kVp increases the beam quality
    C. **True** – increasing peak kVp increases the mean beam energy
    D. **True** – reducing the voltage ripple increases average beam energy and improves beam quality
    E. **False** – appropriate filtration increases beam quality

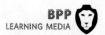

12. X-ray beam intensity
   A. Refers only to the number of photons produced
   B. Is approximately proportional to kV^2
   C. Is directly proportional to mAs
   D. Is unaffected by beam filtration
   E. Is unaffected by voltage waveform

If a point source produces photons, then the number of photons from that source passing through unit area is called the photon fluence. These photons will all have varying energies and the sum of these energies per unit area is called energy fluence. The beam intensity is the energy fluence per unit time.

$$\text{Intensity} = \frac{\text{No. of photons per unit area} \times \text{mean photon energy}}{\text{Unit time}}$$

Beam intensity is directly related to the tube current (the number of electrons flowing from the cathode to the anode) and the exposure time; therefore beam intensity is directly related to mAs. It is approximately proportional to kV^2 but at lower voltages it is closer to kV^3. Since filtration will absorb some of the photons the intensity will decrease. Other factors that will affect the intensity include the voltage waveform (increased intensity with lower waveform ripple) and distance from the anode focal spot (inverse square law).

---

12. A. **False** – it is energy fluence per unit time
   B. **True** – it is approximately equal to kV^2
   C. **True** – beam intensity is directly proportional to mAs
   D. **False** – it will be affected by filtration
   E. **False** – lower voltage waveform ripple increases intensity

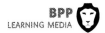

13. A three-phase generator has the following advantages over a single-phase generator
    A. It has a lower voltage waveform ripple
    B. Reduced dose to the patient
    C. Longer exposure times are needed for same film blackening
    D. Higher peak voltage
    E. Does not require rectification

Three phase generators receive current from three different lines. These current sources are 120^0 out of phase with each other. Rectification of this supply will give either a 6-pulse or a 12-pulse voltage waveform (dependent on the degree of rectification that is performed); the 6-pulse having 14% voltage waveform ripple and the 12-pulse having 4% voltage waveform ripple. A single-phase supply has 100% ripple after rectification. Since the three-phase supply provides a much more constant supply, the quality of the X-ray beam produced is increased. This means that shorter exposure times are needed for three-phase supplies, the patient dose is reduced and the penetrating power of the beam is increased.

13. A. **True** – this is an advantage over a single phase supply
    B. **True** – improved beam penetration and shorter exposure times
    C. **False** – shorter exposure times are needed
    D. **False** – if the same voltage is used for both systems the peak voltage will not be different
    E. **False** – rectification is required

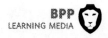

14. Concerning X-ray beam filtration
    A. It occurs at the glass window of general X-ray tubes
    B. Beryllium may be used in mammography X-ray tubes
    C. Filtration will always reduce X-ray output (other factors constant)
    D. Filters are designed solely to stop high energy photons
    E. The K-edge for molybdenum is approx. 30 keV

X-ray beam filtration occurs in all X-ray tubes as the beam passes through the window. It is often quoted in terms of mm of aluminium. The inherent filtration that occurs with diagnostic tubes is approximately 0.5–1 mm of aluminium. In general radiographic machines this is negligible and so extra filters may be required. These are used to absorb the low energy Bremssrahlung radiation, as this is mainly absorbed by the patient and hence increases patient dose whilst contributing little to the image.

In general radiology units the total filtration should be at least 2.5 mm of aluminium (or equivalent). For high kV techniques (chest radiography, etc) further filtration may be needed and a combination filter of aluminium and copper is used. Molybdenum may be used as a filter in mammography units. It has a K-edge of approx. 20 keV. It will be used in conjunction with a molybdenum anode.

It is important to remember that filters will **not** affect the maximum energy of the X-ray spectrum but **will** affect the mean energy of the beam. They will also increase the half-value layer for a particular material.

14. A. **True** – some beam filtration will occur at the window
    B. **True** – a beryllium window is used in mammography units
    C. **True** – any filter will decrease output
    D. **False** – filters are designed to reduce lower energy photons that increase dose
    E. **False** – approximately 20 keV

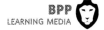

15. Beam hardening
    A. Occurs after filtration
    B. Results in increased penetrating power of the beam
    C. Lowers the maximum photon energy of the beam
    D. Has no effect on the mean energy of the X-ray beam
    E. Lowers the half-value layer (HVL)

After filtration the lower energy photons are removed. Thus the mean energy of the beam is increased but the maximum energy of the photons in the beam remains unchanged. 'Beam hardening' refers to this preferential loss of lower energy photons. Since the mean energy of the beam is increased, the penetrating power of the beam is increased and so is the half value layer (HVL). HVL is defined as that thickness of a given material that will reduce the intensity of a radiation beam to one half of its original value. Beam hardening does **not** occur with monochromatic beams.

15. A. **True** – beam hardening does occur after filtration
    B. **True** – the mean energy is increased and so is the HVL
    C. **False** – the maximum energy of the beam is unaffected
    D. **False** – the mean energy of the beam is increased
    E. **False** – the HVL is increased

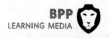

16. With regard to unwanted radiation from an X-ray tube
A. Leakage radiation is the sum of the stray and scattered radiations
B. The tube housing eliminates all unwanted radiation
C. Leakage radiation should be < 1 mGy/hr at 1 m from the focus
D. Increasing the tube kV will increase the amount of scattered radiation in the forward direction
E. Scattered radiation is primarily caused by photoelectric interactions

Unwanted radiation from a source is made up of scattered radiation and leakage radiation. Leakage radiation is that which is transmitted through the tube housing. The components of the housing and the lead lining all help to minimise it, but it is not completely eliminated. It is currently recommended that leakage radiation from the tube does not exceed 1 mGy per hour at a distance of 1 m from the focus.

Scattered radiation is that which has changed direction after leaving the tube. It can be scattered in the patient, at the couch, at the receptor, etc. The sum of leakage and scattered radiation equals stray radiation. Scatter occurs because of Compton interactions more so than photoelectric interactions. Coherent (also called Rayleigh) interactions will also produce scatter but to a much lesser degree. At higher kV the amount of radiation travelling in the forward direction will increase. There will also be a concomitant increase in the amount of forward scatter.

16. A. **False** – leakage radiation is transmitted through the tube housing
B. **False** – it does not eliminate all unwanted radiation
C. **True** – this is a standard requirement
D. **True** – increasing the kV increases the amount of forward scatter
E. **False** – Compton is primarily involved

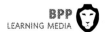

17. Concerning the anode heel effect
    A. It is caused by varying attenuation of the beam within the cathode
    B. It has no practical use
    C. It is related to the target angle
    D. It can be compensated for with the use of filters
    E. It causes the beam intensity to vary but not the beam hardness

---

The anode heel effect causes an asymmetry in the production of X-rays. It is caused by the fact that X-rays produced by interactions deep in the anode are attenuated more by the anode as they travel through it than those which are produced by interactions nearer the surface. The heel effect only occurs along the anode/cathode line. The variation in beam attenuation causes the beam to change in hardness and intensity, and results in higher X-ray intensity at the cathode end and lower X-ray intensity at the anode end. The heel effect varies with the target angle. Decreasing the target angle decreases the spread of the beam and so restricts the field of view.

The heel effect is used in mammography. The higher beam intensity on the cathode side is directed towards the chest wall where greater penetration is required. Some compensation for the heel effect can be achieved by tilting the filter so that different parts of the beam pass through different amounts of the filter.

---

17. A. **False** – varying attenuation in the anode
    B. **False** – it can be used, and is readily used in mammography
    C. **True** – the heel effect varies with the target angle
    D. **True** – filters can be used to compensate for the heel effect
    E. **False** – both the beam intensity and hardness vary

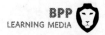

18. The heel effect can be minimised
     A. By increasing the target angle
     B. Using a tungsten/rhenium alloy instead of pure tungsten
     C. Using a smaller field size
     D. Using shorter source-to-film distances
     E. Using tilted filters

The heel effect can be useful as well as detrimental. It is used in mammography. In other situations it may be necessary to minimise its effects. Increasing the target angle will reduce its effects, as will using a smaller field size, where there is a decreased area over which the variation is detected and only the central portion of the beam is utilised. Using a longer source-to-film distance reduces the heel effect because only the central portion of the beam is used. Tilted filters are also used to attenuate the heel effect.

18. A. **True** – increasing the target angle will minimise the heel effect
     B. **False** – this will not affect the heel effect
     C. **True** – a smaller field size will reduce the heel effect
     D. **False** – using a longer source-to-film distance minimises the heel effect
     E. **True** – tilted filters can be used to minimise the heel effect

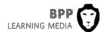

19. The heat loading of an X-ray tube
    A. Is measured in Joules
    B. Is measured in Heat Units
    C. Is always equal to kV × mAs
    D. Is independent of the voltage waveform
    E. Is directly related to the exposure time

The heat rating of an X-ray tube is a measure of the amount of energy that is deposited during an exposure. For constant potential or three-phase supplies it equals kV × mAs. For single-phase supply it is approximately 0.7 x kV × mAs. It is measured in Joules or Heat Units (the old nomenclature) and 1J = 1.4 HU. Since it is a measure of the amount of energy deposited during an exposure it will be related to:

- Tube voltage
- Voltage waveform
- Tube current
- Number of exposures
- Exposure time

19. A. **True** – Joules or Heat Units are used
    B. **True** – Joules or Heat Units are used
    C. **False** – it is kV × mAs for constant potential or three-phase supply only
    D. **False** – it is dependent on the voltage waveform
    E. **True** – it is directly related to the exposure time

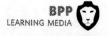

20. Tube rating may be increased by the following
   A. Decreasing the diameter of a rotating anode
   B. Using a rotating anode instead of a stationary anode
   C. Increasing the focal spot size
   D. Using high speed rotating anodes
   E. Using active cooling methods

The tube rating is based on the maximum allowable kilowatts for an exposure time of 0.1 seconds. So the things that will affect heat production (heat loading) will also affect the tube rating. Some of these include:

- Increasing the size of the focal spot so heat is deposited over a larger area
- Using rotating anodes, as this effectively increases the area over which heat is generated
- Increasing the speed of rotation (up to a point) as this will result in increased area for heat deposition and more even heat spread
- Shortening the exposure time
- Increasing the diameter of the rotating anode
- Using active cooling methods. These may be employed in some modern angiography systems and those that require prolonged exposure times.

Obviously, since tube rating is calculated from the kV and mA (for 0.1 sec) both of these will be important with regard to the tube rating.

---

20. A. **False** – increasing the diameter will increase the tube rating
    B. **True** – using a rotating anode effectively increases the size of the focal spot
    C. **True** – increasing the focal spot size deposits heat over a larger area
    D. **True** – increasing the speed increases the area for heat deposition
    E. **True** – allows improved dissipation of heat

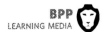

21. Concerning bremsstrahlung radiation
    A. It is caused by electron – electron interactions
    B. It is limited by the filament current
    C. The maximum wavelength is related to the kVp
    D. Account for the majority of X-ray produced in a X-ray tube
    E. Bremsstrahlung X-ray production is higher for tungsten than for molybdenum if all other factors are equal

Bremsstrahlung radiation (braking radiation) is caused by the interaction between electrons (from the cathode) and the nuclei of the atoms that make up the anode. The electrostatic forces between the incoming electrons and the nuclei cause the electrons to change direction, and in the process they lose energy. This loss of energy is released as X-rays.

The low-energy cut-off for these X-rays is because of the heavy attenuation low-energy X-rays undergo as they exit the tube. The high-energy cut-off is because the maximum energy of the X-rays can only be equal to the maximum amount of energy the bombarding electrons had. So if the kVp is 120 kV, then an electron can have maximum 120 keV energy and hence, by the principle of energy conservation, the highest energy an emergent X-ray can have is 120 keV. The high-energy cut-off is therefore limited by the maximum tube potential and not the filament current. The minimum wavelength of the X-rays corresponds with the maximum energy since:

$$\text{Wavelength} = hc/e$$

(where h is Planck's constant, c is the speed of light and e is the energy of electrons.)

The skewed shape of the spectrum is because of the attenuation the X-rays undergo and the fact they are not all produced at the anode surface. Bremsstrahlung radiation accounts for the majority of X-rays produced. Atoms with higher atomic numbers produce

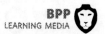

more bremsstrahlung radiation because of the stronger force between the electron and the nucleus.

---

21. A. **False** – caused by interactions between electrons and the anode nuclei
    B. **False** – it is limited by the kV not the current
    C. **False** – the minimum wavelength is related to the kVp
    D. **True** – they account for the majority of X-rays produced
    E. **True** – since the atomic number for tungsten is higher than molybdenum

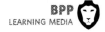

> 22. Concerning the spectrum of radiation produced by an X-ray tube
>
>   A. It is not affected by the anode material
>   B. The minimum X-ray photon frequency is directly related to the maximum tube potential
>   C. The tube current alters the shape of the spectrum
>   D. Increasing tube potential alters the quality of the X-ray spectrum
>   E. The characteristic K-shell radiation energy for tungsten is 69.5 keV

The spectrum of radiation produced is related to both the tube potential and the anode material. These things alter the quality of the X-rays, ie they change the shape of the spectrum. Factors such as exposure time and tube current will alter the number of X-rays produced, and hence change the quantity, but they do not alter the shape of the spectrum. The maximum tube potential is related to the minimum X-ray wavelength and hence the maximum frequency (as wavelength and frequency are inversely related to each other).

---

22. A. **False** – the anode material affects the radiation spectrum
    B. **False** – they are inversely related
    C. **False** – alters the quantity of X-rays but not the spectrum
    D. **True** – tube potential alters the spectrum of radiation produced
    E. **True** – characteristic radiation for tungsten is 69.5 keV

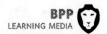

23. The characteristic X-rays produced by an X-ray tube
    A. Contribute significantly more X-rays than bremsstrahlung
    B. Occur at 17.4 keV and 19.6 keV for molybdenum
    C. Are caused by the interaction of bombarding electrons with unbound electrons in the anode
    D. K-shell characteristic X-rays for tungsten will be emitted if the tube potential is set to 60 kV
    E. L-shell characteristic X-rays are useful in general radiology

Characteristic X-rays occur when a bound electron (in the anode) is ejected by a bombarding electron from the cathode. In order to do this the incident electron must have energy greater than the binding energy of the anode electron. It follows that in order to eject an electron from the K shell, an incident electron must have greater energy than the binding energy of the K shell.

Once the electron is ejected, the vacancy it creates needs to be filled. The electron that fills this vacancy may come from a neighbouring shell, eg the L-shell (most likely transition) or even from a free electron. The different characteristic spectral lines are caused by this fact. For example the K-series of lines for tungsten range from 58.5 keV (if the vacancy is filled by a neighbouring L-shell electron) up to 69.5 keV (if a free electron occupies the vacancy).

The vacancies created by the incident electrons can happen in any of the electron shells, with a similar process to the one described earlier occurring afterwards. However, since the binding energy of the other shells is lower, the X-rays produced are of lower energy and are generally absorbed at the tube window, filter etc.

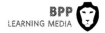

23.　A.　**False** – bremsstrahlung contribute more than characteristic radiation

　　B.　**True** – 17.4 keV and 19.6 keV for molybdenum

　　C.　**False** – characteristic radiation occurs when a bound electron in the anode is ejected by a bombarding electron

　　D.　**False** – K-shell characteristic X-rays will not be produced as the energy requirement is 69.5 keV

　　E.　**False** – The L-shell energies are too low to be practically useful

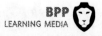

24. With regard to the shape of the X-ray spectrum
    A. Increasing tube current alters the shape of the spectrum
    B. Increasing the exposure time alters the shape of the spectrum
    C. Increasing the kVp above the K-shell binding energy will cause new characteristic X-ray lines to appear on the spectrum
    D. Increasing the kVp shifts the spectrum upwards and towards the right
    E. The characteristic X-ray lines occur at lower photon energy for lower atomic number anodes

The shape of the X-ray spectrum is changed by the kVp. Increasing the kVp will shift the spectrum upwards and to the right. Changing the tube current and the exposure time will not affect the shape of the spectrum; however, they will cause an increase in the amount of bremsstrahlung and characteristic radiation. Obviously no new characteristic lines will appear if the kVp is increased above the K-shell binding energy, as this is the innermost shell of electrons.

24. A. **False** – this alters the quantity of X-rays produced
    B. **False** – no affect on the shape of the spectrum
    C. **False** – this represents the innermost shell of electrons, therefore no new characteristic radiation will appear
    D. **True** – increasing the kVp will shift the spectrum to the right
    E. **True** – since the K-shell binding energies are lower

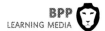

25. The maximum energy of the X-ray photons in a spectrum
    A. Is directly related to the kVp
    B. Is affected by the anode material
    C. Is unrelated to the distance between the anode and the cathode
    D. Is affected by the voltage waveform
    E. Is of the order of 120–140 keV for CT

The maximum energy of the emitted X-ray photons in a spectrum is related to the kVp. It is unaffected by anode material, anode-cathode distance, voltage waveform (notice that the question specifies **maximum** energy). CT uses high energy X-rays and this order of magnitude is correct.

25. A. **True** – the maximum energy is directly related to kVp
    B. **False** – the maximum energy of the photons is not affected by the anode material
    C. **True** – there is no relation between the maximum photon energy and the distance between the anode and cathode
    D. **False** – the mean energy is affected but the maximum energy is not
    E. **True** – this is the standard range for CT

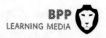

Chapter 3

X-ray
interactions

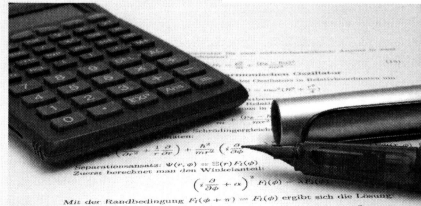

X-ray interactions

Please answer all questions true or false. There is no negative marking.

---

1. The following occur in diagnostic radiology
    A. Compton interactions
    B. Photoelectric interactions
    C. Pair production
    D. Photodisintegration
    E. Rayleigh interaction

As X-ray photons pass through matter they can be attenuated. Attenuation is the sum of scatter and absorption. These processes occur to varying degrees dependent on tissue density, structure, photon energy, etc. Compton, coherent and photoelectric interactions all occur in radiology. Pair production is used in nuclear imaging. Photo-disintegration is important in radiotherapy. In photo-disintegration, a very high energy photon (above approximately 15 MeV) is absorbed by a nucleus which results in immediate disintegration of the nucleus.

---

1. A. **True** – occur in diagnostic radiology
    B. **True** – occur in diagnostic radiology
    C. **True** – occurs in nuclear imaging
    D. **False** – these interactions do not occur in diagnostic radiology
    E. **True** – occur in diagnostic radiology

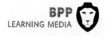

2. Concerning photoelectric effect
    A. Photoelectric effect occurs between photons and free electrons
    B. The incoming photon is completely absorbed
    C. A positive ion is formed in the process
    D. A photoelectron is emitted in the process
    E. The probability of a photoelectric interaction is completely independent of the atomic number of the element

The photoelectric effect occurs when an incident photon interacts with a tightly bound electron. The incident photon is completely absorbed in the process and an electron, termed the photoelectron, is ejected from the atom. This results in the formation of a positive charge ion. The photoelectron then dissipates energy to the surrounding matter by ionisation. These interactions all contribute to patient dose. The probability of a photoelectric interaction is proportional to Z^3/E^3.

2. A. **False** – occurs between photon and tightly bound electron
    B. **True** – the incident photon is completely absorbed
    C. **True** – an electron is ejected resulting in a positive ion
    D. **True** – the ejected electron is termed the photoelectron
    E. **False** – the probability is related to the atomic number of the element

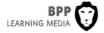

3. The probability of a photoelectric interaction
   A. Is higher for inner shell electrons
   B. Is inversely proportional to Z
   C. Is directly related to E^3
   D. Is inversely proportional to f^3
   E. Continues to increase as the photon energy rises above the K edge

The probability of a photoelectric (PE) interaction occurring is related to:

$$PE\ probability = Z^3/E^3$$

Since $E = hf$, then $E^3 = (hf)^3$, so probability is inversely proportional to f^3.

Therefore, as the atomic number of the material increases the probability of PE interaction also increases. The reverse is true for increasing the incident photon energy. In order for the PE effect to occur, the incident photon must have energy at least equal to the binding energy of the electron. If the incident photon energy was less than the binding energy the electron would not be ejected.

The probability of PE interaction increases as the energy of the photon approaches that of the binding energy of the electron. The probability of the interaction is greatest when the photon energy is just above the binding energy of the electron.

As the photon energy continues to rise the probability decreases. The reason for this is a resonance-like phenomenon and the fact that as the photon energy approaches the binding energy of a new orbit, more electrons become available to undergo PE interactions. For these reasons the PE effect is most likely to occur with K-shell electrons (as long as the incident photon energy exceeds the K-binding energy.) Approximately 80% of PE interactions occur with K-shell electrons.

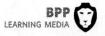

3. A. **True** – it is higher for inner shell electrons
    B. **False** – it is proportional to Z
    C. **False** – it is inversely related to E^3
    D. **True** – it is inversely proportional to f^3
    E. **False** – it does not continue to rise above the K edge but rather decreases

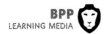

4.   Regarding coherent scatter
     A.   It results in absorption
     B.   It accounts for approximately 5–10% of total
          interactions in diagnostic radiology
     C.   It is more likely to occur with high atomic number
          elements
     D.   It is more likely to occur with increasing incident
          photon energy
     E.   It does not contribute to the dose a patient
          receives

Coherent scatter, also called Rayleigh scatter, occurs when photons excite an atom but pass straight through it. The photon causes the electrons to vibrate at a frequency corresponding to that of the photon. The electron then dissipates this energy in all directions. There is no energy deposition and so there is no dose to the patient. This is a cause of scatter without energy loss.

The electrons involved in the process must remain bound, and so it is favoured by electrons with high binding energies, ie atoms with high Z. Conversely, the energy of the photon could be low and so it is more likely with low-energy beams.

Coherent scatter is proportional to Z^2/E.

4.   A.   **False** – there is no absorption
     B.   **True** – it accounts for a minority of interactions
     C.   **True** – it is more likely with high Z
     D.   **False** – more likely with lower energy beams since it is
                     inversely proportional to E
     E.   **True** – energy is not deposited so there is no dose to
                     the patient

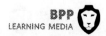

5. With regard to beam attenuation
   A. Scatter is the sole cause of beam attenuation
   B. Absorption is important for image contrast
   C. Beam attenuation can result in characteristic radiation production
   D. Mono-energetic beams undergo beam hardening
   E. X-ray photons may pass through matter without attenuation

Attenuation is the sum of scatter and absorption. It is possible for X-ray photons to pass through matter without any attenuation. This is referred to as penetration.

In plain film radiography, absorption increases image contrast but also increases patient dose. Scatter results in some contribution to patient dose but degrades the image. As poly-energetic/polychromatic beams pass through matter there is a change in the spectrum of the beam due to selective attenuation of certain X-ray photons (lower-energy photons). This results in beam hardening. With mono-energetic beams this does not occur – put simply, the beam will either be stopped or it will not. Beam attenuation is caused by the interaction of the X-ray photons with the matter via several different interactions, eg photoelectric, Compton, elastic/coherent/Rayleigh, pair production and photo-disintegration. Characteristic radiation may be produced in photoelectric interactions and so beam attenuation can result in characteristic radiation production.

5. A. **False** – absorption is also a cause of attenuation
   B. **True** – this is the basis of radiological imaging
   C. **True** – characteristic radiation can be produced by photoelectric interactions
   D. **False** – poly-energetic beams undergo beam hardening
   E. **True** – this is called penetration

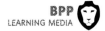

6. In Compton interactions
   A. Photons interact with inner shell electrons
   B. The loss of energy by the scattered photon is dependent on the incident photon energy
   C. The process is one of partial absorption and scatter
   D. All the energy of the incident photon can be transferred to the recoil electron
   E. Increasing the incident photon energy results in a decreased proportion of energy going to scatter

Compton interactions occur between an incident photon and an outer shell electron. These loosely bound electrons can be thought of as free electrons since the difference between their binding energy and the energy of the incident photon is so great. The Compton interaction can be thought of as an inelastic reaction.

The photon strikes the electron and this results in a scattered photon with lower energy. It also results in a Compton electron/recoil electron. The recoil electron is responsible for increasing patient dose and the scattered photon is the cause of scatter. Hence the interaction is one of partial absorption and scatter. Since there is always a recoil electron and a scattered photon in the process not all the energy can be transferred from the incident photon to the recoil electron.

It can be shown that the energy lost by the incident photon is related to its original energy. So if a photon is scattered by 60° the proportion of energy taken by the recoil electron at 20 keV is 2% but at 1 MeV it is 50%. Hence, at higher incident photon energy there is a decreased proportion of energy going to scatter and more going to absorption.

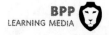

6. A. **False** – occurs between incident photon and outer shell electron
    B. **True** – at increased incident photon energy there is a decreased proportion of energy going to scatter
    C. **True** – the interaction is of scatter and absorption
    D. **False** – some of the energy has to go to the scattered photon
    E. **True** – increased photon energy results in decreased scatter and more absorption

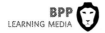

7. The Compton effect
    A. Is the most common interaction in diagnostic radiology
    B. Is proportional to the number of electrons in a material
    C. In biological tissues Compton interactions are heavily dependent upon atomic number
    D. A positron is produced
    E. Dominates in water at 45 keV

The Compton effect is the most common interaction process at diagnostic energy levels. For soft tissue at approximately 25–30 keV the Compton and PE effects are equal in magnitude. With increasing energy the probability of Compton interactions is related to $1/E$ but for PE it is $1/E^3$. Compton interactions are between incident photons and 'free' electrons. The Compton effect is proportional to the number of electrons in a material but for most biological tissues the electron density (number of electrons divided by atomic mass) is approximately constant at around 0.5. The exception to this is hydrogen that has an electron density of 1. Hence tissues rich in hydrogen show increased Compton reactions.

7. A. **True** – it is most common at diagnostic radiology energy levels
    B. **True** – it is proportional to the number of electrons
    C. **False** – the electron density is relatively constant in biological tissues
    D. **False** – a positron is not produced in Compton interactions
    E. **True** – more common at this energy level

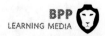

8. The linear attenuation co-efficient
   A. Only takes into account Compton interactions
   B. Is independent of incident photon energy
   C. Increasing physical density generally increases the linear attenuation co-efficient (LAC)
   D. Is independent of kV but is dependent on mAs
   E. Is measured in cm^2

The linear attenuation co-efficient (LAC) is the proportion of photons that are lost from the beam as they travel a unit distance in a material. It is measured in cm^{-1} or mm^{-1}, not cm^2. It is a cumulative score and it takes into account the sum of all the different types of interaction that can occur between photons and matter, ie Compton, photoelectric, coherent, etc. Since the LAC is related to the interactions between photons and matter, and these interactions are dependent on energy the LAC is related to incident photon energy. Generally the LAC decreases with increasing photon energy **except** at K-edges. It also generally increases with increasing density.

8. A. **False** – it is a cumulative score and takes account of all interactions
   B. **False** – the LAC is energy dependant
   C. **True** – generally increases with density
   D. **False** – dependent on kV but not on mAs
   E. **False** – measured in cm^{-1} or mm^{-1}

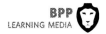

9. Factors that increase the linear attenuation co-efficient (when all other variables remain constant) include
    A. Increasing the atomic number of the material
    B. Increasing the maximum kVp of the tube
    C. Increasing the density of the matter
    D. Increasing the distance between the source and the object
    E. Increasing the tube mA

The linear attenuation co-efficient is a property of a material. The things that cause it to increase are an increase in density of the material and increasing the atomic number of the material. Increasing the incident photon energy will result in decreased attenuation; hence increasing the tube kV causes a reduction in the attenuation. Altering the mA has no effect.

9. A. **True** – this causes an increase in the LAC
    B. **False** – causes a decrease in the LAC
    C. **True** – increases the LAC
    D. **False** – no effect
    E. **False** – no effect

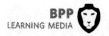

10. With regard to the half-value layer
    A. It is the same as the linear attenuation co-efficient
    B. It is inversely related to the mass-attenuation co-efficient
    C. It represents the thickness of material required to attenuate a mono-energetic beam by 50%
    D. It is not dependent on incident photon energy
    E. At 100 keV the half-value layer (HVL) is higher for muscle than bone

---

The half-value layer is another term used to quantify beam penetration. It is used for poly-energetic beams whereas the linear and mass attenuation co-efficient are used for mono-energetic beams. It is inversely related to the linear attenuation co-efficient and is approximately calculated as follows:

$$HVL = 0.693/\text{linear attenuation co-efficient}$$

Therefore, anything that affects the linear attenuation co-efficient will also alter the HVL. Since increasing material density causes an increase in the LAC, this will cause a decrease in the HVL (from the above equation) so at 100 keV the HVL for bone is less than for muscle (approximately 2.3 cm for bone, compared to 3.9 cm for muscle).

---

10. A. **False** – the HVL is inversely related to the LAC
    B. **False** – it is inversely related to the LAC not the MAC
    C. **False** – HVL is relevant to polyenergetic beams not monoenergetic beams
    D. **False** – it is dependent on incident photon energy
    E. **True** – since the density of muscle is less than bone

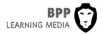

11. Concerning the interactions of X-ray beams with matter
   A. Back scatter generally carries more energy than scatter in the forward direction
   B. Increasing the tube kV results in a more penetrating beam
   C. Increasing the tube kV increases the HVL for a given material
   D. The HVL is not altered by beam hardening
   E. A steady increase in the photon energy causes a steady reduction in the attenuation of a beam

Scatter caused by X-ray interactions can travel in any direction. The scatter that travels in a forward direction has more energy, in general, than scatter travelling backwards. Increasing the photon energy will cause more scatter to travel in a forward direction. Increasing the tube kV increases the penetrating power of the beam. This means the half value layer of a material also increases (and the LAC decreases). However, increasing the photon energy does not mean that the attenuation changes steadily because of K-edges. This principle is important with regard to filters, contrast agents, etc. Also, since a beam becomes more penetrating as it travels through a material (lower energy photons are attenuated) the HVL of the beam will change.

11. A. **False** – scatter forward carries a greater energy generally
     B. **True** – increasing the kV increases the penetration and hence increases the HVL
     C. **True** – the HVL will increase with increased kV
     D. **False** – beam hardening will alter the HVL since the beam becomes more penetrating
     E. **False** – this is not the case because of K-edges

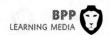

12. The half-value layer for muscle is 39 mm at 100 keV. Therefore
    A. At 50 keV the HVL would be greater than 39 mm
    B. The 100 keV beam will be attenuated by 50% after travelling through 39 mm of muscle tissue
    C. At 200 keV the linear attenuation co-efficient will be less than the linear attenuation co-efficient at 100 keV
    D. Bone will have a lower HVL at 100 keV
    E. After 78 mm the beam would be attenuated by 66%

If the HVL for bone at 100 keV is 39 mm then after this distance the beam is attenuated by 50%. This is the definition of HVL. Increasing the photon energy will cause the LAC to reduce but the HVL to increase (they have an inverse relationship). Decreasing the photon energy will increase the LAC and hence reduce the HVL. After 78 mm, the beam will be reduced by approximately 75%–50% by the first HVL then 50% again in the second HVL (50% of 50%) hence 75%. This is not technically correct since the second HVL will be slightly different to the first but without further information you cannot calculate the exact beam attenuation.

The HVL of bone will be lower because of its increased atomic number and density.

12. A. **False** – decreasing the photon energy will decrease the HVL
    B. **True** – this is the definition of the HVL
    C. **True** – increasing the photon energy will decrease the LAC
    D. **True** – bone has a higher density and atomic number than muscle so will have a lower HVL
    E. **False** – it will be attenuated by close to 75%

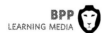

13. The mass attenuation co-efficient (MAC)
      A.   Is related to the linear attenuation co-efficient
      B.   Is not interchangeable with the LAC
      C.   Is independent of the density of a material
      D.   Has units of cm^{-1}
      E.   Attenuation of the beam can be calculated as the product of the MAC and the mass thickness

---

The mass attenuation co-efficient (MAC) is the linear attenuation co-efficient (LAC) divided by the density of the material through which the beam passes. As such it is independent of the density of a material whereas the LAC is not. It is measured in units of cm^2/kg or cm^2/g. Whilst the MAC and the LAC are related they are not interchangeable. To calculate the attenuation of a beam the mass thickness of a material must be known. This is measured in g/cm^2 or kg/cm^2. The product of the mass thickness and MAC is the attenuation of the beam.

---

13. A.   **True** – the MAC is the LAC divided by the density of the material
      B.   **True** – they are not interchangeable
      C.   **True** – the MAC is independent of the density
      D.   **False** – it has units of cm^2/kg or cm^2/g
      E.   **True** – the product of the MAC and mass thickness is the attenuation of the beam

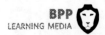

14. Practical uses of the linear attenuation co-efficient
     A. Calculating Hounsfield units in CT
     B. Assigning colour scales in nuclear imaging techniques
     C. Calculating the half-value layer of a beam
     D. Determining the thickness of barium plaster required in an interventional radiology suite
     E. Calculating the thickness of lead shielding required for adequate thyroid protection

The LAC determines the fraction of photons removed from a beam travelling unit distance through a medium. Practical applications include calculating HVL, determining how thick a material will be needed to provide adequate shielding and assigning Hounsfield units in CT.

14. A. **True** – this is one of the uses
     B. **False** – this is not dependent on the LAC
     C. **True** – since they are related
     D. **True** – used to determine the adequate shielding thickness
     E. **True** – used to determine the adequate shielding thickness

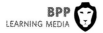

15. At 50 keV the following are true
    A. Compton interactions predominate in soft tissue
    B. Pair production accounts for approximately 10% of interactions
    C. The K-edge for iodine is approached
    D. The energy of photons scattered by Compton interaction through 90° and 180° is approximately the same
    E. The point at which Compton interactions predominate over PE interactions for aluminium is at approximately 50 keV

Interactions in matter are dependent upon photon energy. PE pre-dominates at lower energies and Compton at higher energies. At 50 keV the Compton process is more important in soft-tissue. In aluminium this energy is approximately where the PE and Compton processes are equal (higher Z). As photon energies change the probability of interactions changes, and this is the cause of K-edges (as explained earlier). The K-edge for Iodine is 33 keV. It has Z of 53.

Compton interactions produce scatter. As the photon energy increases an increasing proportion of the scattered photons travel in a forward direction. The energy carried by the scattered photons changes dependent on the incident photon energy. As the angle of deflection increases, the energy retained by the scattered photon decreases. At 50 keV the energy carried by a photon scattered through 90° is approximately equal to a photon scattered by 180°.

15. A. **True** – these interactions predominate at 50 keV in soft tissue
    B. **False** – coherent (Rayleigh) interactions account for 5–10% of interactions
    C. **False** – the K-edge for iodine is 33 keV
    D. **True** – at 50 keV this statement is true
    E. **True** – in aluminium, Compton and PE interactions are approximately equal at 50 keV

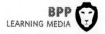

Chapter 4

Film-screen radiography

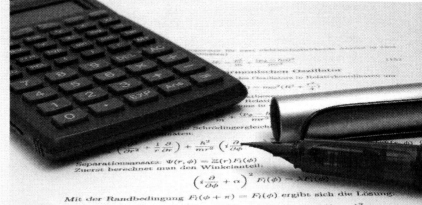

Film-screen radiography

Please answer all questions true or false. There is no negative marking.

1.　Regarding radiographic film
    A.　Film consists of a photographic emulsion base with a polyester coating
    B.　The emulsion is a suspension of silver bromide crystals
    C.　Each crystal is roughly 1 μm in size
    D.　Photographic emulsion is much more sensitive to ultraviolet light than X-ray
    E.　When a crystal absorbs a photon it allows a bromide ion to move to a sensitivity speck

---

Film consists of a polyester base normally covered on both sides with a photographic emulsion. The emulsion contains a suspension of silver halide crystals, which are normally silver iodobromide crystals (90% bromide, 10% iodide). Each crystal is roughly 1 μm in size, the polyester base is 0.2 mm thick and the emulsion is 5–10 μm thick. Photographic emulsion is much more sensitive to both visible and ultraviolet light than X-rays. When a light photon is absorbed in the crystal the energy allows an electron to travel to a sensitivity speck. When enough of these accumulate a silver ion is attracted to neutralise the electron so forming a microscopic speck of silver at this site, making up the latent image in the photographic emulsion.

1.　A.　**False** – film consists of a polyester emulsion base with a emulsion coating
　　B.　**False** – the emulsion is a suspension of silver halide crystals
　　C.　**True** – each crystal is roughly 1 μm in size
　　D.　**True** – photographic emulsion is much more sensitive to ultraviolet light than X-ray
　　E.　**False** – when a crystal absorbs a photon it allows a electron to move to a sensitivity speck

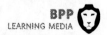

2. Which of the following statements regarding film processing are correct
   A. The first stage of processing of a film is development by an acidic solution
   B. Film developer contains a reducing agent
   C. Crystals with no latent image are unaffected by the developer
   D. The film is washed in an alkaline solution
   E. Washing helps prevent the film turning yellow with age

Processing of the film involves three stages. The film first needs to be developed, using an alkaline solution that contains a reducing agent which enters the crystal at the site of the latent image to turn the silver ions into atoms, hence forming silver grains on the film surface. This process preferentially occurs on crystals with a latent image; however if the film is exposed to the developer too long or at the wrong temperature or strength it will begin to affect the unexposed crystals. The next stage in processing is to fix the film with an acidic solution of thiosulphate. This removes the remainder of unaffected silver ions, hence stopping the emulsion from any further photographic reaction with light. The final stage is to wash the film in water, removing the fixing solution which stops the film turning yellow/brown with age.

---

2. A. **False** – the first stage of processing of a film is development by an alkaline solution
   B. **True** – film developer contains a reducing agent
   C. **False** – even crystals with no latent image will eventually be affected by the developer
   D. **False** – the film is washed in water
   E. **True** – washing helps prevent the film turning yellow with age

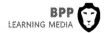

3. With regard to the optical density
   A. Optical density is defined as the ratio of transmitted light to incident light
   B. If 10% of light is transmitted the optical density is 0.1
   C. If the film has a double-sided emulsion the average of the density through both is calculated
   D. A density of above 3 is too dark to be viewed properly
   E. Optical density is measured with a sensitometer

Optical density is defined as the log of the ratios of the incident to transmitted light. Hence if 10% of the incident light is transmitted the optical density is 1. If 0.1% of the incident light is transmitted the optical density would be 3. When a double-sided photographic emulsion is used the optical densities are added together. Generally an adequate optical density of a properly exposed film is roughly around 1 although it can be slightly higher. Normally an optical density of over 3 is considered too dark to be adequately viewed. Optical density can be calculated by a densitometer. This is a machine that contains a light source and a light detector and measures the ratio of transmitted and incident light through a film.

3. A. **False** – optical density is defined as the log of the ratios of incident to transmitted light
   B. **False** – if 10% of light is transmitted the optical density is 1
   C. **False** – if the film has a double-sided emulsion the total density through both is calculated
   D. **True** – a density of above 3 is too dark to be viewed properly
   E. **False** – optical density is measured with a densitometer

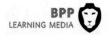

4. Intensifying screens have the following properties
   A. The polyester base is roughly 0.25 mm thick
   B. The polyester base is covered with a photographic emulsion
   C. Rare earth materials such as calcium tungstate are commonly used in the phosphor
   D. A double-coated X-ray film normally uses two screens
   E. The screen converts X-rays into visible light

Photographic emulsion is much more sensitive to visible and ultraviolet light than X-rays. Film screens are used to increase the efficiency of X-rays by converting them into visible light, hence reducing the amount of ionising radiation required to give an adequate image. Screens are comprised of a 0.25 mm polyester base that is covered with a 0.1–0.5 mm layer of phosphor crystals. These phosphor crystals absorb the X-ray photons and re-emit the energy as visible light. The traditional phosphor used was calcium tungstate. However, this has been mostly replaced by rare earth materials such as gadolinium oxysulphide, as this is more efficient. A double-coated emulsion film commonly uses two intensifying screens either side of the film, the rear screen exposing the rear emulsion.

4. A. **True** – the polyester base is roughly 0.25 mm thick
   B. **False** – the polyester base is covered with a layer of phosphor crystals
   C. **False** – calcium tungstate is not considered a rare earth material
   D. **True** – a double-coated X-ray film normally uses two screens
   E. **True** – the screen converts X-rays into visible light

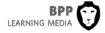

> 5. Intensifying screen phosphors have which of the following properties
>   A. Calcium tungstate has a K-edge at 70 keV
>   B. Lanthanum oxybromide has a K-edge above that of calcium tungstate
>   C. Calcium tungstate emits a green light
>   D. Lanthanum oxysulphide emits a blue light
>   E. Gadolinium oxysulphide can only be used with an orthochromatic film

Calcium tungstate has a K-edge at roughly 70 keV whilst the characteristic radiation peaks of tungsten (the most common target material used in X-ray tubes) are 58 keV and 68 keV. This means the absorption offered by the 70 keV K-edge is not ideal, with poor absorption of the characteristic radiation peaks. Rare earth materials have generally superseded calcium tungstate as a screen phosphor as their K-edge is better matched, having lower K-edges between 57–70 keV. Rare earth materials are also more efficient at converting X-rays into visible and ultraviolet light. Different phosphors emit different spectrums of visible and ultraviolet light and need different films. Calcium tungstate (which emits violet and blue light) and lanthanum oxybromide (which emits blue light) can be used with normal X-ray film (sensitive to ultraviolet and blue light only). Lanthanum and gadolinium oxysulphide (which emit green light) must be used with an orthochromatic film.

---

5. A. **True** – calcium tungstate has a K-edge at 70 keV
   B. **False** – lanthanum oxybromide has a K-edge below that of calcium tungstate
   C. **False** – calcium tungstate emits a violet and blue light
   D. **False** – lanthanum oxysulphide emits a green light
   E. **True** – gadolinium oxysulphide can only be used with an orthochromatic film

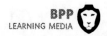

6.   Which of the following regarding the characteristic curve
      are correct
      A. The characteristic curve describes the response of
          log exposure against log optical density
      B. The characteristic curve is derived by a sensitometer
      C. The toe region describes the high exposure shallow
          part of the curve
      D. At very high exposures the optical density will rise
          again after the slope has already reached a plateau
      E. An unexposed film has an optical density of zero

The characteristic curve describes the response of a film-screen combination to X-rays and is plotted on a graph as log exposure against optical density. The curve is derived by a sensitometer, a small machine that has a light source and filters allowing a series of different exposures to be compared on film, which mimics a film-screen exposed to a variety of radiation exposures.

The curve classically has three distinct parts, the toe region at low exposure and optical density which has a shallow slope; the shoulder region at high exposure and optical density with a shallow curve reaching a plateau; and the area of correct exposure in between, where the curve rises most steeply. The toe region does not actually begin at an optical density of zero, as the curve takes into account the fog and base levels; hence even unexposed film does not have an optical density of zero. The curve forms a plateau at the shoulder region; however with very high exposures solarisation occurs causing a loss in optical density.

6.   A. **False** – the characteristic curve describes the response
              of log exposure against optical density
      B. **True** – the characteristic curve is derived by a
              sensitometer
      C. **False** – the toe region describes the low exposure shallow
              part of the curve
      D. **False** – very high exposures cause a loss in optical density
              after the slope has already reached a plateau
      E. **False** – fog and base levels mean the optical density is
              never zero

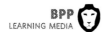

7. Regarding base, fog and speed
    A. Base level is increased when the film base absorbs a greater proportion of light
    B. Fog level is increased when the silver halide crystals acquire a latent image due to manufacturing technique
    C. Base plus fog in a well developed film normally has an optical density of 0.5–1.0
    D. Speed of the film is defined as the reciprocal of the exposure needed to produce a film density of 1
    E. A decrease in the average crystal size in the film causes a decrease in the speed

The base level represents the intrinsic optical density which occurs from the silver halide crystals acquiring a latent image during manufacture and the film base itself absorbing light at the time of viewing. The fog level represents the optical density acquired from storage and by processing conditions. Normally the base plus fog is in the range of 0.15–0.2 in a well developed film. The speed of the film is the reciprocal of the exposure needed to produce a film optical density of base + fog + 1. Film speed increases with the average size of the emulsion crystals as larger crystals require less light to form latent images within them.

7. A. **True** – base level is increased when the film base absorbs a greater proportion of light
    B. **False** – base level is increased when the silver halide crystals acquire a latent image due to manufacturing technique
    C. **False** – base plus fog in a well developed film normally has an optical density of 0.15–0.2
    D. **False** – speed of the film is defined as the reciprocal of the exposure needed to produce a film optical density of base + fog + 1
    E. **True** – a decrease in the average crystal size in the film causes an increase in the speed

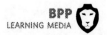

8. Which of the following regarding film gamma and latitude are correct
    A. Film gamma depends on the average size of the crystals
    B. The greater the film gamma the greater the contrast
    C. Film latitude is increased by a greater gamma
    D. The higher the film gamma is, the easier it is to interpret a plain X-ray film
    E. The film latitude describes the range of densities between exposures of 0.25 and 2

Film gamma is the average slope of the characteristic curve in the region of correct exposure, typically describing the curve between optical densities of 0.25 and 2. The range of exposures that give these optical densities is known as the latitude. The greater the film gamma the greater the film contrast and hence the smaller the film latitude; however with too high a film contrast (and hence small latitude) fine detail may be lost. The film gamma depends on the range of crystal sizes, not their average size, as the bigger the range of crystal size, the wider the variety of response to light. Hence, the greater the range of exposures needed to produce an image, causing the film gamma to be shallower.

---

8. A. **False** – film gamma depends on the range of the size of the crystals
    B. **True** – the greater the film gamma the greater the contrast
    C. **False** – film latitude is decreased by a greater gamma
    D. **False** – if the film gamma is too high fine detail may be lost
    E. **False** – the film latitude describes the range of densities between optical densities of 0.25 and 2

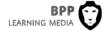

9. Variation in the developing conditions will result in which of the following
   A. Increasing the developer temperature initially causes the speed to increase
   B. Increasing the developer concentration increases the base level
   C. Increasing the developing time above recommendations causes the gamma to decrease
   D. Developing conditions are optimised for minimum fog and gamma
   E. Increasing the developer concentration above recommendations can cause the optical density to fall

Developing conditions are optimised to give maximum gamma and minimum fog levels. Increasing the developer temperature and concentration normally increases the rate of reaction, increasing the speed and initially the gamma but also increasing the fog level. The base level is not affected by the developer concentration. Gamma levels initially increase with high temperatures and concentrations, but beyond a certain point the fog level rises so much that the gamma effectively decreases.

9. A. **True** – increasing the developer temperature initially causes the speed to increase
   B. **False** – increasing the developer concentration increases the fog
   C. **True** – increasing the developing time above recommendations causes the gamma to decrease
   D. **False** – developing conditions are optimised for minimum fog and maximum gamma
   E. **False** – increasing the developer concentration above recommendations can cause the gamma to fall

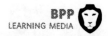

10. Regarding intensification factor and speed class
A. Intensification factor is defined as the air kerma required to make the optical density 1
B. Intensification factor is normally in the range of 30–100
C. Speed is normally defined as 1000/K where K is the air kerma in µGy needed to give an optical density of 1
D. If the speed classification is 250 the air kerma for a satisfactory exposed radiograph is 4µGy
E. Rare earth film-screen combinations normally have a speed in the region of 400

The intensification factor describes how the film-screen reduces the X-ray exposure compared to film alone. It is defined as the ratio of air kerma required to make the optical density 1 for film, compared to the air kerma required to make the optical density 1 with a film-screen combination. Normal film-screen intensification factors are in the region of 30–100. The speed class of a film-screen combination is defined as 1000/air kerma (µGy) required to give a film optical density of 1 + base + fog. Hence if the air kerma for a film-screen combination was 4 µGy, then the speed class would be 1000/4 = 250. A normal film-earth screen combination is in the region of 400.

---

10. A. **False** – intensification factor is defined as the ratio of air kerma required to make the optical density 1 for film compared to a film-screen combination
B. **True** – intensification factor is normally in the range of 30–100
C. **False** – speed is normally defined as 1000/K where K is the air kerma in µGy needed to give an optical density of 1 + base + fog
D. **True** – if the speed classification is 250 the air kerma for a satisfactory exposed radiograph is 4 µGy
E. **True** – rare earth film-screen combinations normally have a speed in the region of 400

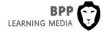

11. With regard to contrast, which of the following statements are true?
   A. With respect to film-screen radiography, contrast is defined as the difference in optical density between two areas
   B. There is an inverse relationship between contrast and gamma
   C. High levels of ambient light when viewing film normally increases the contrast
   D. There is an inverse relationship between contrast and film latitude
   E. High levels of contrast cause loss of fine detail when viewing a film

---

Contrast is defined as the difference in optical density between two corresponding areas. If film gamma increases then the change in optical density for a given change in exposure will be greater, hence contrast will increase. Similarly, if the latitude is greater then the film gamma must decrease so contrast would decrease.

A higher contrast level causes more polarisation of the colour towards one end of the black-white film spectrum, hence fine detail may be lost. Even if the film contrast is optimised it should also be noted that the reporting conditions will again affect the contrast with high levels of ambient light reducing the level of contrast the eye can perceive.

---

11.   A. **True** – with respect to film-screen radiography, contrast is defined as the difference in optical density between two areas
      B. **False** – if the gamma is higher then the contrast will be greater
      C. **False** – high levels of ambient light when viewing film normally decrease the contrast
      D. **True** – there is an inverse relationship between contrast and latitude
      E. **True** – high levels of contrast cause loss of fine detail when viewing a film

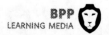

12. Regarding screen unsharpness
    A. Increasing the screen phosphor thickness increases unsharpness
    B. The sooner the X-ray photon interacts with the front screen phosphor the less the blurring
    C. The thicker the screen phosphor the greater the speed of the film-screen combination
    D. Increasing the screen phosphor thickness causes an increase in noise
    E. Increasing the screen phosphor efficiency causes an increase in noise

In a film-screen combination the properties of the phosphor can greater affect the sharpness of the end film. Ultraviolet and visible light is emitted from the phosphor in all directions, hence the closer it does this to the photographic film emulsion the less the light spreads. Therefore, in the front screen the sooner the X-ray interacts with the phosphor the more the ultraviolet and visible light can spread and the more blurring there is. Similarly, making the phosphor layer thicker will increase the blurring. Increasing the phosphor thickness will also mean a greater proportion of X-ray photons passing through are absorbed into the phosphor crystal layer, increasing the efficiency and hence the speed.

Noise is produced when fewer photons are responsible for making up the picture. If the phosphor layer increases, although more X-ray photons are absorbed compared to a thinner phosphor, the actual number of X-ray photons needed to produce an adequately exposed film is the same (though the radiation dose to the patient is less), so there is no effect on noise. However if the phosphor is more efficient (hence it is better at amplifying the X-ray signal) then less photons are needed to create an adequately exposed film so the noise is greater.

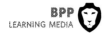

12. A. **True** – increasing the screen phosphor thickness increases unsharpness
     B. **False** – the later the X-ray photon interacts with the front screen phosphor, the less the blurring
     C. **True** – the thicker the screen phosphor the greater the speed of the film-screen combination
     D. **False** – increasing the screen phosphor thickness causes no effect on noise
     E. **True** – increasing the screen phosphor efficiency causes an increase in noise

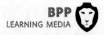

13. Regarding screen unsharpness
  A. Adding a reflective layer to the screen base will increase both the efficiency and unsharpness of the film-screen combination
  B. Coloured dyes allow a better absorption of X-rays in the phosphor, increasing efficiency
  C. Poor film-screen contact will cause an increase in blurring
  D. 'Crossover' describes blurring caused by divergence of the X-ray beam as it crosses from the front to rear emulsion
  E. Total unsharpness is derived from the square root of the sum of the geometric, movement and screen unsharpness

---

A reflective layer is sometimes added to the base to reflect any ultraviolet or visible light which may emit from the phosphor away from the surface of the film and bounce it back towards the film. This increases the efficiency of the phosphor. However, as the photons are travelling further when in the phosphor they also diverge more, hence increasing the blurring.

Coloured dyes can be used to absorb light as it passes through the phosphor. Light emitted from the phosphor which takes a wide divergence travels further before it reaches the film and hence is more likely to be absorbed by the dyes. This decreases the blurring but also decreases the sensitivity.

If there is a gap between the film and the screen this will cause increased divergence of the light, again increasing blurring.

Crossover occurs when light emitted from the phosphor crosses through the front emulsion, through the base and reacts in the rear emulsion, or visa versa, leading to increased divergence and more blurring. As X-ray beams also diverge the image on the rear emulsion will be slightly larger than the front emulsion, an effect known as parallax.

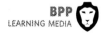

Screen unsharpness is only one of three factors contributing to overall unsharpness including geometric and movement unsharpness. Total unsharpness is defined as the square root of the sum of the squared geometric, movement, and screen unsharpness.

---

13. A. **True** – adding a reflective layer to the screen base will increase both the efficiency and unsharpness of the film-screen combination

B. **False** – coloured dyes allow a better absorption of light in the phosphor increasing efficiency

C. **True** – poor film-screen contact will cause an increase in blurring

D. **False** – parallax describes blurring caused by divergence of the X-ray beam as it crosses from the front to rear emulsion

E. **False** – total unsharpness is derived from the square root of the sum of the squared geometric, movement and screen unsharpness

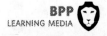

Chapter 5

Factors affecting the radiological image

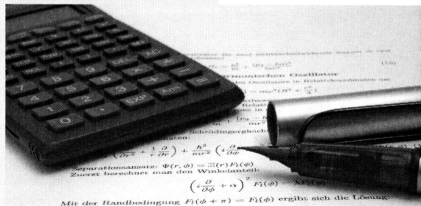

Factors affecting the radiological image

Please answer all questions true or false. There is no negative marking.

> 1. The following techniques can be used to minimise scatter
>   A. Using collimation
>   B. Air gaps between the focus and the object
>   C. Intensifying screens
>   D. Using compression
>   E. Increasing the tube kV

Scatter is undesirable as it reduces subject contrast. It results from Compton interactions. Reducing scatter will improve the final image contrast. There are several ways in which scatter can be reduced.

Collimation of the beam decreases the total mass irradiated, therefore there is less tissue in which interactions can occur.

Lower kVp promotes photo-electric interactions. This is limited by the fact that at lower kV patient penetration may be inadequate and film blackening may be sub-optimal.

Using an air gap between the object and the film can reduce scatter because there is less chance the scattered radiation will reach the film.

Anti-scatter grids are the most effective way to remove scattered radiation.

Compression of the patient forces tissue out of the primary beam, hence there is less tissue for interactions.

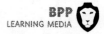

1. A. **True** – collimation is used to decrease scatter
   B. **False** – the air gap should be between the object and the film in order to reduce scatter
   C. **False** – intensifying screens do not minimize scatter
   D. **True** – compression decreases the number of interactions and hence reduces scatter
   E. **False** – lowering the kV promotes photoelectric interactions

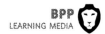

2. The effect of Compton scatter on the final image can be reduced by
    A. Decreasing the kV but increasing the mAs to optimise the film blackening
    B. Using a lead-backed cassette
    C. Using a grid with a higher grid ratio
    D. Breath-holding
    E. Increasing the focus-object distance

Using cassettes with a high atomic number backing will reduce backscatter. The interactions that occur in the backing plate will be photoelectric. Grids can be used to reduce scatter. The grid ratio is defined as:

Strip height/distance between the lead strips

Increasing the grid ratio will result in less scattered radiation reaching the film. Decreasing the kV will increase photo-electric interactions and decrease Compton interactions. Altering the mA will not affect the probability of either Compton or photo-electric interactions but it is required to maintain film blackening. Breath-holding will not reduce Compton scatter. Instead, it will reduce motion blur.

Increasing the focus-object distance will not alter Compton interactions. The air gap needs to be introduced between the object and the film.

2. A. **True** – lowering the kV promotes photoelectric interaction
    B. **True** – using lead-backed cassettes helps to reduce backscatter
    C. **True** – grids minimize scatter and higher grid ratio decreases the scatter
    D. **False** – this reduces motion blur
    E. **False** – this will not effect Compton interactions

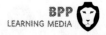

3. Anti-scatter grids
   A. Are placed behind the patient and the film
   B. Are composed of alternating bands of two different high atomic number materials
   C. Where focused, must be placed at the correct distance
   D. Must be placed parallel to the direction of the beam
   E. Cause an increase in dose

Anti-scatter grids are an effective and commonly used way of decreasing scatter. They are placed between the object and the film perpendicular to the beam. The 'holes' need to be parallel to the central ray of the beam. They are made up of many strips of highly attenuating material (eg lead). The X-ray photons pass through the 'holes' between the lead strips that are filled with low-attenuating material.

The grid ratio is the ratio of the height of the lead strips to the distance between them. Increasing the grid ratio will decrease the amount of scattered ratio reaching the film. However, it will also decrease the amount of primary radiation reaching the film. Hence, to maintain film blackening the exposure must be increased, resulting in increased patient dose.

Many different types of grid are available. Focused grids have diverging strips and they must be used at specific focal distances to prevent inappropriate absorption of the primary beam.

3. A. **False** – grids are placed between the patient and the film
   B. **False** – they are made of alternating high and low attenuating materials
   C. **True** – if an inappropriate distance is used with focused grids there will be absorption of the primary beam and the scatter
   D. **False** – grids are placed perpendicular to the beam
   E. **True** – grids increase dose to patients

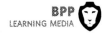

4. Regarding the movement of anti-scatter grids
   A. It is generally oscillatory
   B. The grid may be seen on the final image if it is stationary
   C. The movement only needs to occur during the exposure
   D. Mobile X-ray units often use stationary grids
   E. With single-phase X-ray units the movement of the grid must coincide with the X-ray pulse

Stationary grids can be seen as fine lines on the final image. This effect can be overcome by moving the grid. Generally the motion is oscillatory in nature and it starts before the exposure and continues after the exposure. The device that moves the grid is called a Bucky (after its inventor). In single-phase X-ray units the timing of the grid movement must not coincide with that of the pulses otherwise it will appear as if the grid is stationary (a stroboscopic effect). This is not required in medium or high-phase systems. Mobile units will often use stationary grids with low grid ratios.

4. A. **True** – oscillating motion is commonly used
    B. **True** – grids will be seen as fine lines on the image if they are stationary
    C. **False** – the movement usually starts before and stops after the exposure
    D. **True** – mobile units often use stationary grids with low grid ratios
    E. **False** – the grid movement must not coincide with the pulses

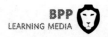

5. With linear focused grids
    A. Decentring produces generally lighter films
    B. As the amount of decentring increases the film becomes lighter
    C. Placing the grid upside down will produce a wide exposed area
    D. Use of the wrong focus-film distance does not affect the central portion of the film
    E. They are commonly used in extremity radiography

Linear focused grids have their lead strips progressively angled on moving away from the central axis. The grid must be faced the correct way, and be at the correct distance from the focus. If the distance is wrong the central portion of the film will be exposed but there will be a progressive increase in the cut-off towards the edge of the film. Decentring tends to produce a overall lighter film. This increases with increasing decentring.

As mentioned earlier, grids are not used for all types of radiographs. They are not required for most extremity radiography.

---

5. A. **True** – decentring produces lighter films
    B. **True** – increasing the decentring makes the film lighter
    C. **False** – if the grid is upside down a narrow exposed area is seen with very little blackening either side
    D. **True** – the central portion will not be affected
    E. **False** – they are generally not required for extremity radiography

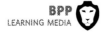

> 6. The modulation transfer function (MTF)
>   A. Is based on Fourier analysis
>   B. Is used to describe the resolution capability of an imaging system
>   C. Only the film has an MTF
>   D. The MTF can never exceed 1.0
>   E. At high spatial frequencies the MTF is close to 1

The modulation transfer function (MTF) is a curve based on Fourier analysis that is used to describe the resolution capability of an imaging system. It is a ratio of the output to the input signal amplitude in a given imaging system for each spatial frequency. At high spatial frequencies the MTF falls towards 0. This corresponds to poor visibility of small structures. At low spatial frequencies the MTF is closer to 1, and represents the ability to clearly visualise large structures. Digital systems can have an MTF above 1 through the use of edge enhancement and other such technology. Each component within an imaging system has it own MTF.

6. A. **True** – it is based on Fourier analysis
    B. **True** – the MTF describes the resolution capability
    C. **False** – every component in an imaging system has an MTF
    D. **False** – the MTF can exceed 1 in digital systems
    E. **False** – the MTF falls towards 0 at high spatial frequencies

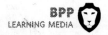

7. With regard to the modulation transfer function
   A. It is derived from the line spread function
   B. A two-dimensional Fourier transformation is used on the line spread function
   C. The MTF of a system is the product of the MTF for all the individual components
   D. The limiting MTF is caused by the individual component with the highest MTF
   E. The MTF falls towards 0 with increasing spatial frequency

---

The MTF is derived from the line spread function. It is a one-dimensional Fourier analysis of the line spread function. Each component in an imaging system has its own MTF. The overall MTF for an imaging system is the product of these individual MTFs. Hence, the overall MTF will be limited by the component with the lowest MTF in the system. The MTF tends to fall towards 0 as the spatial resolution of objects increases.

---

7. A. **True** – it is a one-dimensional Fourier transformation of the line spread function
   B. **False** – a one-dimensional Fourier transform is used
   C. **True** – the MTF of a imaging system is the product of the MTF for each component part
   D. **False** – the limiting MTF is caused by the lowest MTF in the system
   E. **True** – the MTF falls towards 0 with higher spatial frequency

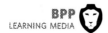

> 8. The following are true regarding the MTF (at a given spatial frequency)
>   A. The MTF for non-screen film is higher than for screened film if other variables are constant
>   B. Movement unsharpness does not change the MTF
>   C. Increasing the size of the focal spot will decrease the MTF
>   D. Increasing the magnification will increase the MTF
>   E. In screen-film radiography the screen has the lower MTF

At a given spatial frequency the following are true:

- Movement unsharpness will degrade the MTF
- Increasing the size of the focal spot will degrade the MTF (due to geometric reasons)
- Magnification will degrade the MTF (due to geometric reasons)
- Screens degrade the MTF because of spread of light in the screen
- Screens have a lower MTF than film
- Fast screen-films have lower MTF than slow screen-film

8. A. **True** – screens degrade the MTF
   B. **False** – movement unsharpness degrades the MTF
   C. **True** – larger focal spots degrade the MTF
   D. **False** – magnification degrades the MTF
   E. **True** – screens have a lower MTF than film

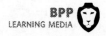

9.   Which of the following affect geometric unsharpness?
      A.   Focus-film distance
      B.   Object-film distance
      C.   The target angle
      D.   The tube anode-cathode distance
      E.   The size of the actual focal spot

Geometric unsharpness is caused by the fact that the actual focal spot is a finite size. The penumbra is given by the equation:

$$b \sin a \{d/ (FFD-d)\}$$

where:
b = actual focal spot size
a = target angle
d = object to film distance
FFD = focus to film distance

Hence it can be seen that anything that affects the magnification or the focal spot size causes a change in the geometric unsharpness.

---

9.   A.   **True** – focus-film distance alters unsharpness
      B.   **True** – object-film distance alters unsharpness
      C.   **True** – the target angle alters unsharpness
      D.   **False** – this has no effect on unsharpness
      E.   **True** – the actual focal spot size alters the unsharpness

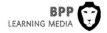

10. The following will result in increased geometric unsharpness
   A. Introducing an air gap where there previously was none
   B. Using macro-radiographic techniques
   C. Increasing the exposure time
   D. Increasing the tube kVp
   E. Changing the target angle from 6° to 20°

Changing the exposure time may affect movement unsharpness. Changing the tube kVp can change movement unsharpness by altering the exposure time and it can also affect edge unsharpness. It will not affect the geometric unsharpness. All the other factors will change the factors influencing geometric unsharpness.

---

10. A. **True** – this affects the object-film distance
   B. **True** – macro-radiographic techniques alter geometric unsharpness
   C. **False** – this increases motion blur
   D. **False** – this will not alter geometric unsharpness
   E. **True** – changing the target angle alters geometric unsharpness

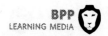

11. Motion blur can be minimized by
   A. Increasing the tube current
   B. Shortening the exposure time
   C. Using a slower film-screen combination
   D. Magnification of the image
   E. Using compression paddles in mammography

Motion blur can be caused by voluntary or involuntary motion. The main factors that determine the degree of motion blur are the speed at which the underlying tissue is moving and the exposure time. Decreasing the underlying movement can only be done to a certain degree, eg immobilisation devices such as paddles in mammography. Decreasing the exposure time can be achieved in a variety of ways including:

• Increasing the mAs
• Using a faster film-screen combination
• Using multiple sources, eg 256 slice CT scanners compared with 4 slice

11. A. **True** – this will minimize exposure time
    B. **True** – shortening the exposure time will minimize motion blur
    C. **False** – fast film-screen combination minimizes motion blur
    D. **False** – magnification will magnify any blur
    E. **True** – this minimizes movement

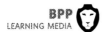

12. The following factors will increase unsharpness (other variables constant)
   A. Smaller focal spot size
   B. Longer exposure time
   C. Double emulsion films
   D. Increased screen thickness
   E. Long object to film distance

Smaller focal spots will decrease geometric unsharpness whereas longer object to film distances will increase it. Longer exposure times will increase motion blur. Double emulsion films will cause parallax. Increasing the screen thickness will allow more light diffusion within the screen.

---

12. A. **False** – larger focal spot sizes increase unsharpness
   B. **True** – longer exposure time will increase movement unsharpness
   C. **True** – double emulsion films cause parallax
   D. **True** – increased screen thickness increases unsharpness
   E. **True** – this increases geometric unsharpness

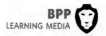

13. Regarding screen blur
   A. It is caused by light diffusion in the film
   B. Thin screens have better spatial resolution than thick screens
   C. Thick screens have poorer absorption efficiencies than thin screens
   D. Poor film–screen contact does not affect screen blur
   E. Parallax errors are seen in single emulsion films

Screen blur is caused by the diffusion of light within the screen. This diffusion decreases the MTF at a given spatial resolution compared to a film without a screen. Thick screens have a higher absorption efficiency and so are faster (therefore will reduce motion blur, dose to the patient etc.) but they allow more diffusion of light compared to thin screens. Thin screens, on the other hand, allow less diffusion of light and so have better spatial resolution but they have poor absorption efficiency (they are slow screens and so cause more movement unsharpness, increased dose to the patient, etc.) Good contact between the screen and the film is required to prevent increased blur. Parallax errors are only seen in double emulsion films.

13. A. **False** – screen blur is caused by the diffusion within the screen
    B. **True** – less diffusion occurs in thin screens, therefore they have better spatial resolution
    C. **False** – thick screens have higher absorption efficiencies
    D. **False** – increased blur occurs with poor screen-film contact
    E. **False** – parallax error is seen in double emulsion films

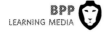

14. Regarding screen/film speed and noise (for a fixed optical density)
    A. Faster films tend to produce more noise
    B. Thicker screens increase noise
    C. Screens with a high conversion efficiency tend to produce less noise for the same optical density
    D. Screen/film speed can be increased with a lower number of detected X-rays photons
    E. Increasing the number of detected photons increases the noise

Noise is related to the number of photons detected. In screen/film combinations the screen absorbs the X-ray photon and then re-emits light photons. Screen/film speed can be increased by using screens with higher conversion efficiency. However, since fewer X-ray photons are required to produce the same number of light photons, and hence optical density, the noise is increased. So, faster films and screens with higher conversion efficiency produce more noise. Thicker screens have higher absorption efficiency and so stop more incoming photons. However, they do not have higher conversion efficiency so they do not cause an increase in the noise – it remains the same.

14. A. **True** – faster film produce more noise
    B. **False** – thicker screens decrease noise
    C. **False** – higher conversion efficiency produce more noise for the same optical density
    D. **True** – they have higher conversion efficiency
    E. **False** – this decreases the noise

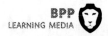

Chapter 6

Image intensifiers and fluoroscopy

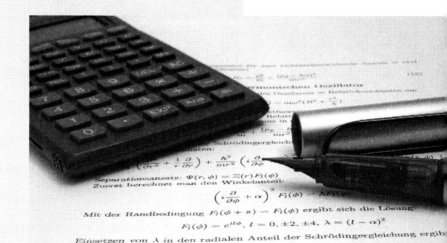

Image intensifiers and fluoroscopy

Please answer all questions true or false. There is no negative marking.

1. Regarding image intensifier phosphors
   A. The input phosphor absorbs incoming X-rays and converts them to electrons
   B. The input phosphor is typically 2.5 cm in diameter
   C. The output phosphor is typically zinc cadmium sulphide activated with silver
   D. Glass lenses are used to focus the image onto the output phosphor
   E. The input phosphor is typically 200–400 μm thick

Image intensifiers use a combination of input and output phosphors, accelerating anodes and lenses to produce an image. The input phosphor is usually made of caesium iodide and typically has a thickness of 200–400 μm. It is larger than the output phosphor and is often approximately 25 cm in diameter. At the input side of the image intensifier the X-ray first passes through a thin layer of aluminium before hitting the input phosphor. The input phosphor converts the X-ray into light photons which are emitted. These then strike a photocathode that absorbs the light photons and emits electrons that strike the output phosphor. The output phosphor is often made of zinc cadmium sulphide activated with silver. For a 25 cm input phosphor a 2.5 cm output phosphor is often used.

1. A. **False** – it converts incoming X-rays into light photons
   B. **False** – the output phosphor is 2.5 cm in diameter
   C. **True** – the output phosphor is zinc cadmium activated with silver
   D. **False** – several electrodes in the shape of metal rings act to focus the image onto the output phosphor
   E. **True** – the input phosphor is typically 200–400 μm thick

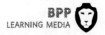

2. Image intensifier artefacts
   A. Lag is of major concern in modern caesium iodide units
   B. Lag is typically 1 ms for modern CsI units
   C. Pincushion artefacts are produced by all image intensifiers
   D. The brightness at the centre is less than the periphery
   E. Straight lines may appear curved on the final image

Image intensifiers suffer from a range of artefacts. Lag is when there is continued luminescence at the output phosphor after the X-rays at the input phosphor has stopped. It typically results in around 1 ms delay and is often of little importance in modern units. Straight lines can indeed appear curved and this is called the pincushion distortion. All image intensifiers produce this artefact. Vignetting is the change in brightness across the image – brighter in the centre than at the edges.

---

2. A. **False** – lag is not of major importance in modern units
   B. **True** – in modern units lag is approximately 1 ms
   C. **True** – all image intensifiers produce pincushion distortion
   D. **False** – brightness is higher at the centre
   E. **True** – this is pincushion distortion

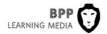

3.	Image intensifier tubes
	A.	Contain a vacuum
	B.	Have a potential difference across the tube of 25–35 keV
	C.	Use electrodes to focus the electrons produced at the photocathode
	D.	The anode of an image intensifier is the aluminium coating on the output phosphor
	E.	Changing the position of the electrodes allows magnification

---

The image intensifier tube contains a vacuum. At one end is the input screen and at the opposite is the output screen. There is a potential difference of 25–35 keV between the input and output screens. The cathode is the photocathode and the anode is the aluminium coating on the output screen. The potential difference is responsible for accelerating the electrons towards the anode and it is responsible for the flux gain in the image intensifier. Several metal rings in the image intensifier are responsible for focusing the electrons produced. Electromagnetic forces produced by the electrodes constrain the electrons on certain paths. By altering the force exerted by them, the focus (crossover point of the electrons) can be moved nearer the output screen and this is what causes image magnification.

3.	A.	**True** – image intensifiers contain a vacuum
	B.	**True** – the potential difference between input and output screens is 25–35 keV
	C.	**True** – electrodes in the shape of rings focus the electrons
	D.	**True** – the aluminium coating acts as the anode
	E.	**False** – changing the electromagnetic force produced by the electrodes allows magnification

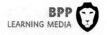

4. Concerning image intensifier gain
   A. The gain of an image intensifier system is only caused by minifying the image
   B. The potential difference between the cathode and the anode has no effect on the overall gain of the system
   C. Magnification reduces the brightness at the output phosphor in systems that do not use automatic brightness control
   D. Gain of a system reduces over time
   E. Overall brightness gain is 5000–10000

The overall gain in the image intensifier system is called the brightness gain. it is the product of minification gain and flux gain. minification gain is equal to the ratio of the areas of the input and output screens for example 25 cm to 2.5 cm diameter $(250/25)^2 = 100$.

After electrons are released from the photocathode they are accelerated across the tube by a potential difference of 25–35 keV. This causes them to increase in energy. When they strike the output phosphor they cause the release of approximately 50–100 photons. Hence each electron releases 50–100 photons at the output phosphor, and this is termed the flux gain.

The brightness gain is then $50 \times 100 = 5000$.

When you magnify the image you are reducing the minification gain. Hence, the brightness of the image decreases in systems that do not use automatic brightness controls. Over time, the gain of an image intensifier system decreases due to loss of detection efficiency at the phosphors.

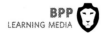

4. A. **False** – gain is a product of minification and flux
    B. **False** – flux gain is related to the potential difference between anode and cathode
    C. **True** – magnification reduces the brightness in systems without automatic brightness control
    D. **True** – efficiency decreases over time and leads to lower gain
    E. **True** – overall gain is around 5000–10000

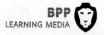

5. The input screen of modern image intensifiers
  A. Use caesium iodide as the input phosphor because it has K-edges at 43 keV and 46 keV
  B. Caesium antimony is used as the photocathode
  C. Caesium iodide has an amorphous structure
  D. The caesium iodide input phosphor layer is 0.1–0.4 mm thick
  E. The thick input phosphor layer causes a significant decrease in the spatial resolution of the system but increases the X-ray detection efficiency to approximately 98%

The input phosphor is usually made of caesium iodide and the photocathode from antimony caesium. The caesium iodide is used as it has K-edges at 33 and 36 keV which increases its absorption efficiency and it can be made into a crystalline structure. The crystals are thin and needle-like with a diameter of about 5 μm. Light reflects internally within the crystals and so there is a minimal spread of light. This means that a thicker crystal can be used without it significantly affecting spatial resolution. The crystal is normally 0.1–0.4 mm thick and this detects about 60% of incoming X-rays.

5. A. **False** – the K-edges for caesium iodide are at 33 and 36 keV
  B. **True** – caesium antimony is used as a photocathode and caesium iodide as an input phosphor
  C. **False** – caesium iodide is laid down in needle-like crystals that acts as light pipes
  D. **True** – the input phosphor is 0.1–0.4 mm thick
  E. **False** – efficiency is approximately 60% and there is not a significant decrease in spatial resolution

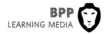

> 6. In fluoroscopy
>   A. In automatic brightness control systems magnification will result in an increased dose to the patient
>   B. The entrance surface dose (ESD) cannot exceed 100 mGy/min
>   C. Pulsed fluoroscopy does not alter the dose to a patient
>   D. Patients receive doses of approximately 10–30 mGy/min
>   E. Continuous fluoroscopy is pulsed at 15–20 pulses/second

Fluoroscopy systems commonly employ methods to automatically maintain brightness levels at the viewing screen. This is achieved by measuring the light intensity at the output screen and then adjusting the kV and/or mA if the brightness changed. Normally the central portion of the image is measured. Various factors will cause the brightness to change, and hence change the kV and/or mA. These factors will then alter the dose to the patient. Magnification is important as it increases the dose to patients. When magnification is performed the brightness gain is decreased because there is loss of the minification gain (remember, brightness gain is the product of flux gain and minification gain). The system will compensate for the loss in brightness by adjusting the kV and/or mA that will result in a higher dose to the patient. Holding the image intensifier away from the patient has a similar effect.

Doses to patient cannot exceed 100 mGy/min and most procedures involve doses of 10–30 mGy/min. Pulsed fluoroscopy is a simple method to reduce the dose. So-called 'continuous' fluoroscopy is actually pulsed fluoroscopy at 25–30 pulses/sec. At this rate the eye cannot discern the difference between pulsed and 'continuous'.

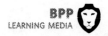

6. A. **True** – automatic brightness control will increase the dose if magnification is used since overall gain (minification gain x flux gain) will go down
    B. **True** – patient dose cannot exceed 100 mGy/min
    C. **False** – pulsed fluoroscopy will help to reduce patient dose
    D. **True** – most procedures will give a patient dose of approximately 10–30 mGy/min
    E. **False** – continuous fluoroscopy is pulsed at 25–30 pulses/sec

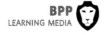

7. Image quality in fluoroscopy
    A. Magnification does not alter spatial resolution
    B. A limiting spatial resolution of 4–5 lp/mm can be expected
    C. Increasing the mA of the system will decrease the noise
    D. The input screen is the 'quantum sink'
    E. Spatial resolution is tested using a Leeds Test Object

In fluoroscopy the limiting spatial resolution is of the order of 4–5 lp/mm. This is slightly improved by using magnification. The spatial resolution in fluoroscopy is principally limited by blurring. Noise is another important feature that will influence contrast resolution and it is due to the low dose rates employed. Noise can be reduced by using higher mA but this will increase the dose to the patient. The quantum sink in the fluoroscopy system is the input screen. After this point no change in the gain will improve the signal to noise ratio. Spatial resolution is tested using a grid Test Object. A Leeds Test Object is used for contrast resolution.

7. A. **False** – magnification slightly improves spatial resolution
    B. **True** – spatial resolution for fluoroscopy is 4–5 lp/mm
    C. **True** – noise can be reduced by increasing mA but this will increase patient dose
    D. **True** – the quantum sink in fluoroscopy units is the input screen
    E. **False** – a Leeds Test Object is used for contrast resolution

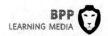

8. Methods used to minimise patient dose in fluoroscopy include
   A. Using magnified views
   B. Frame-grabbing instead of spot-films
   C. Collimation of the image
   D. Holding the image intensifier far from the patient
   E. Using continuous fluoroscopy to decrease the time taken to acquire the necessary images

There are several methods that can be employed to minimise the dose to a patient undergoing a fluoroscopy investigation. Using magnified images increases dose. Frame-grabbing does not increase patient dose, whereas spot-films do. Frame-grabbing involves storing the screening images. A spot-film is a single image that uses high mA to reduce noise. Collimation of the image will help to reduce patient dose. If collimation is used to view the central part of the image then the automatic brightness control will automatically reduce the tube output. This is because the central part of the film is brighter than the periphery. Keeping the image intensifier close to the patient will result in less of an effect from an air gap. Therefore the image will be recorded as being brighter, and so the automatic controls will not activate to increase the tube output. Obviously, using pulsed fluoroscopy will reduce the dose.

8. A. **False** – magnification increases dose in systems that use automatic brightness control
   B. **True** – frame-grabbing helps minimise dose
   C. **True** – collimation helps reduce dose
   D. **False** – the image intensifier should be held close to the patient to minimise dose
   E. **False** – pulsed fluoroscopy should be used to minimise dose

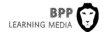

9.   Regarding the use of image intensifiers
      A.   The X-ray tube voltage is between 70 and 90 keV
      B.   Grids are not used in fluoroscopy
      C.   Bandwidth in a TV system determines the horizontal resolution
      D.   High image lag in TV systems results in minimal motion blur
      E.   Low image lag in TV systems results in a reduced SNR

Typical X-ray tube voltages used in fluoroscopy are of 70–90 keV and current of 1–5 mA. The low mA accounts for the low dose but the increase in noise. They do use grids to remove scatter and the grids typically have a grid ratio of 10:1. Televisions are used to watch the images produced during fluoroscopy. They are generally subdivided into two systems:

- Plumbicon – low lag, and so there is less motion blur with movement. However, with low lag there is increased noise because less temporal averaging occurs (multiple images are not 'summed').
- Vidicon – high lag, so there is less noise because many images are 'summed' but motion is not easily followed.

These systems may soon be replaced by CCD TV cameras which have virtually no lag.

9.   A.   **True** – tube voltage is between 70–90 keV
      B.   **False** – grids are used to remove scatter
      C.   **True** – bandwidth determines horizontal resolution
      D.   **False** – low lag allows motion to be followed with minimal motion blur
      E.   **False** – low lag has less motion blur but there is increased noise

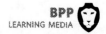

10. Concerning dose in fluoroscopy
   A. A barium enema investigation results in an effective dose of approximately 7 mSv
   B. A dose area product meter is mounted between the patient and the image intensifier
   C. Using a carbon fibre table can help to reduce patient doses
   D. In over-couch fluoroscopic systems a lead skirt attached to the table will help reduce patient doses
   E. A barium swallow is considered a low dose investigation

The doses from fluoroscopic investigations can vary greatly. As with all imaging modalities involving ionising radiation the ALARA principle is paramount. A typical barium enema effective dose is 7–8 mSv. This is considered a high dose investigation (>2 mSv). Barium swallows carry an effective dose of 1.5 mSv and are considered medium dose investigations. Common methods of monitoring patient doses are to use dose area product meters. These are mounted at the tube window and they calculate the total dose over a given area. They are useful to estimate the skin dose. Using carbon fibre tables can help to lower patient dose as there is less attenuation of the beam by the couch. A lead skirt will not minimise patient dose but is a useful way to protect the radiologist from stray radiation.

10. A. **True** – a barium enema results in a dose of 7–8 mSv
   B. **False** – a DAP meter is mounted at the tube window
   C. **True** – carbon fibre couches have a low attenuation and so help reduce patient dose
   D. **False** – a lead skirt helps reduce dose to the radiologist and radiographer
   E. **False** – it is not considered a low dose investigation

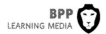

Chapter 7
Mammography

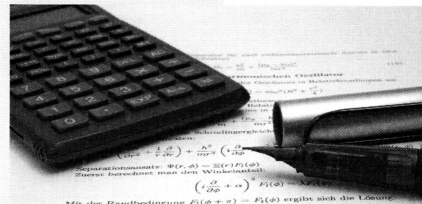

Mammography

Please answer all questions true or false. There is no negative marking.

---

1. Typical features for a dedicated mammography unit include
    A. Tube voltage of 40–50 kVp
    B. Molybdenum target anode
    C. Single-phase voltage supply
    D. Molybdenum window
    E. 0.3 mm focal spot for magnification mammography

Mammography units are dedicated solely for this purpose. They have significantly different operating characteristics to conventional radiology X-ray tubes. Tube voltage is 25–35 kVp and often the target material is molybdenum. Rhodium is also used as the target anode. These produce characteristic X-rays at the optimal energy levels to maximise tissue contrast (approximately 20 keV). Molybdenum characteristic X-rays are produced at 17.9 keV and 19.5 keV. Rhodium characteristic X-rays are produced at 20.2 keV and 22.7 keV – better for penetration of thicker and/or denser breast tissue. In order to produce these characteristic X-rays the operating tube voltage needs to be higher than this. The window of a mammography unit is frequently made of beryllium.

Added filtration is also often used and the material used is dependent on the anode material. Molybdenum filters are used for molybdenum targets and rhodium filters are used for rhodium targets. In each case they have the advantage of filtering the high and low energy radiations but having minimal effect on the characteristic radiations. Therefore they help reduce patient dose (absorbing low energy radiation) and improving contrast (absorbing high energy radiations). They are known as K-edge filters.

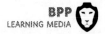

To reduce exposure times three-phase or high frequency generators are used.

---

1. A. **False** – tube voltage is 25–35 kVp
    B. **True** – molybdenum can be used as the target material
    C. **False** – most modern units use triple phase or high frequency voltage supplies
    D. **False** – beryllium is used for the window
    E. **False** – 0.1 mm focal spot is required for magnification mammography

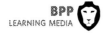

2. In mammography X-ray tubes
   A. The anode is stationary
   B. Exposure times can be up to 4 seconds
   C. The normal focal spot size is 0.3 mm
   D. The anode side of the tube is placed towards the patient
   E. The heel effect is not used in mammography

Mammography tubes use small focal spots and can have quite long exposure times (up to 4 seconds for dense breast tissue). This means that significant heat loading is paced on the anode. Rotating tubes are therefore needed to cope with this stress. In normal mammography a 0.3 mm focal spot is used. In magnification mammography a 0.1 mm focal spot is used. The heel effect is a useful tool in mammography. The increased intensity of the beam on the cathode side can be used to image the tissue near the chest wall. Here the tissue is thicker and so increased penetration is needed. This can be done by placing the cathode side of the tube towards the patient.

---

2. A. **False** – a rotating anode is used
   B. **True** – exposure time can be long for dense tissues and to achieve adequate film blackening
   C. **True** – in normal mammography the focal spot is 0.3 mm (0.1 mm in magnification mammography)
   D. **False** – the cathode side is placed towards the patient
   E. **False** – the heel effect is exploited to penetrate thicker tissue

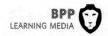

3. Compression in mammography
   A. Usually uses a force of 110–200 N
   B. Must be used for all women
   C. Reduces patient dose
   D. Helps to reduce motion artefact
   E. Results in images being less sharp

Compression is used in mammography since it:

- Reduces patient dose
- Reduces scatter
- Reduces motion artefact
- Increases sharpness
- Spreads the breast tissue and may allow better detection of abnormalities.

The compression is achieved using radio-lucent paddles between which the breast is placed. The force is normally between 110–200 N. It should be used for women that can tolerate it but many find it uncomfortable. Women with very small breasts and/or augmentations will not be suitable for breast compression.

---

3. A. **True** – force is normally between 110–200 N
   B. **False** – not all women require compression
   C. **True** – compression reduces patient dose because less tissue is irradiated
   D. **True** – compression holds the breast still, reducing motion blur
   E. **False** – results in images being more sharp

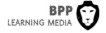

4. Regarding mammography film processing and viewing
   A. Optimal film density is 1.5–2.0
   B. Higher developer temperatures may be used in processing
   C. Films with high gamma are needed
   D. Rare earth screens are not used in mammography
   E. Parallax effects are minimised by using double emulsion films

---

The detection of abnormalities on mammograms is a highly specialised and difficult procedure. The linear attenuation (at 20 keV) co-efficient of fibro-glandular tissue and carcinoma is 0.8 and 0.85 respectively. Hence differences in contrast are subtle and anything that will improve image quality and contrast is essential.

Mammography uses single screens and single emulsions. The single screen helps to improve resolution by limiting diffusion within it. Single emulsion films limit the parallax effect that can occur with dual emulsion films. For contrast to be optimized a high gamma film is needed. The high gamma necessitates a narrow film latitude. The optimal film density is higher than that of conventional radiography – 1.5 to 2.0. This again results in better film contrast. To achieve a higher optical density, higher developer temperatures may be used alongside special processors and prolonged cycle times.

---

4. A. **True** – optimal film density is 1.5 – 2.0
   B. **True** – higher development temperatures may be required to achieve the higher film density
   C. **True** – high gamma films are needed to maximise contrast
   D. **False** – rare earth screens are used eg lanthanium bromide, gadolinium oxysulphide
   E. **False** – parallax effects are minimised by using single emulsion films

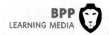

5.   In magnification mammography
      A.   The distance between the X-ray source and the image
            is increased
      B.   0.1 mm focal spot size is commonly used
      C.   A grid is used
      D.   The typical source-to-film distance is about 65 cm
      E.   Scatter is reduced by the use of an air gap

Magnification mammography is achieved by using a stand-off. Here the distance between the source and film are kept constant but the stand-off moves the breast 15–30 cm closer to the source. The magnification effect is therefore equal to the ratio of the focus-film distance to the focus-object distance (FFD/FOD). This is approximately 1.8–2.0 for most mammography units. The stand-off introduces an air-gap that helps to reduce the amount of scatter reaching the film. This means that a grid is no longer required. To increase geometric sharpness a small focal spot is used. The smaller focal spot size means lower mA are required to prevent overheating. To counteract this and achieve optimum film blackening, longer exposure times are used.

---

5.   A.   **False** – the distance between the source and image is
                  kept constant
      B.   **True** – 0.1 mm focal spot size for magnification
                  mammography
      C.   **False** – grids are not used in magnification
                  mammography
      D.   **True** – typical source to film distance is 65 cm
      E.   **True** – an air gap is used to minimise scatter

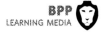

6. Mammograms
   A. Have a limiting spatial resolution of up to 20 lp/mm
   B. Have a film density of 1.5–2.0
   C. Should be viewed on boxes with luminance of 1500 cd/m²
   D. May use terbium activated Gd_2O_2S intensifying screens
   E. Are not affected by quantum mottle

For state-of-the-art systems the spatial resolution can be up to 20 lp/mm. This can be higher in magnification mammography. The major source of noise in film-screen mammography is quantum mottle. In order to maximise contrast the film densities tend to be higher than in conventional radiography. For mammography they are normally 1.5–2.0. The intensifying screens use rare earth metals such as gadolinium. The viewing conditions are very important in mammography because the contrast between normal and abnormal tissue may be very small. It is recommended that films are viewed on boxes with a luminance of 3000 cd/m² and the ambient light is kept to absolute minimum. Hot lights should also be available.

---

6. A. **True** – spatial resolution is up to 20 lp/mm
   B. **True** – film density is 1.5–2.0
   C. **False** – special light boxes with luminance of 3000 cd/m²
   D. **True** – rare earth screens are used including gadolinium oxysulphide
   E. **False** – quantum mottle is the major source of noise in mammography

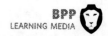

7. Regarding mammography
   A. The photoelectric interaction predominates
   B. Characteristic X-Rays for Mo are 17.9 and 19.5 keV
   C. Tube output is related to kV^2
   D. Beryllium windows are used because of their low attenuation properties
   E. 0.3 mm molybdenum filters are used with Mo anodes

Mammography tubes operate at around 25–35 kVp. At this lower kV the tube output is more closely related to kV^3. In most conventional radiography it is related to kV^2. At the lower energy values photoelectric interactions predominate over Compton scatter. This helps to increase contrast. The window on mammography tubes is often made of beryllium. It has an atomic number of 4 and low attenuation properties. Therefore it does not significantly alter the beam quality. In contrast, K-edge filters are used to alter the beam quality. A molybdenum filter is used in conjunction with a molybdenum anode. This is about 0.03 mm thick.

7. A. **True** – photoelectric effect predominates over Compton in mammography
   B. **True** – the characteristic X-rays of molybdenum are 17.9 and 19.5 keV
   C. **False** – tube output is more closely related to kV^3
   D. **True** – beryllium has low attenuation properties
   E. **False** – a 0.03 mm filter is used

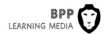

8. Methods used to optimize image quality in mammography include
   A. Breast compression
   B. Use of Al filters
   C. Stationary grids
   D. Dual emulsion films
   E. Films with gamma over 3

Image quality in mammography needs to be excellent. The methods used to optimise image quality are:

- Breast compression – minimises motion, spreads breast tissue, increases geometric sharpness
- Filters are used but these are K-edge filters. They eliminate high energy radiation that would reduce contrast
- Moving grids are used. Carbon fibre is used as the interspace material. Specialised grids used only for mammography have been developed
- Single emulsion films and single screens are used. The screen and emulsion are on the side furthest away from the breast. The single screen helps limit light diffusion within the screen and hence improve resolution. The single emulsion film limits parallax defects
- Films with high gamma (over three) to improve contrast
- Low kVp to allow photoelectric interactions to predominate and maximise contrast.

8. A. **True** – minimises movement and spreads the breast tissue
    B. **False** – Al filters attenuate the low energy beam too much and therefore are not used
    C. **False** – moving grids are used
    D. **False** – single emulsion film is used to minimise parallax effects
    E. **True** – film with high gamma is used to improve contrast

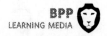

9.   Regarding patient dose in mammography
    A. Grids are used to improve contrast and decrease dose
    B. The Average Glandular Dose is the preferred measurement
    C. Typical dose is 1–5 mGy
    D. For a woman aged 50–65 a mammogram exposure of 2 mGy carries a risk of inducing fatal cancer of 1 in 50000
    E. Filtration has no effect on dose and is used only to improve the quality of the image

Mammography is a screening tool that is performed on many healthy women. The risk-benefit ratio needs to be considered in this situation because of the potential to induce cancer. As such, doses must be kept to an absolute minimum. The Average Glandular Dose is the preferred measurement. For an average mammogram using a grid the dose is in the region of 1.5–3 mGy. At a dose of 2 mGy for a woman aged 50–65 the risk of inducing a fatal cancer is approximately 1 in 50000. Screening programs are expected to reduce the mortality of breast cancers by about 40%. Grids used in mammography behave like grids used in general radiography in that they increase dose to the patient. Filtration helps to reduce dose to the patient by reducing the amount of low energy photons in the spectrum.

9.   A. **False** – grids increase dose
    B. **True** – the Average Glandular Dose is the preferred measurement
    C. **False** – typical dose is 1.5–3 mGy
    D. **True** – a dose of 2 mGy for women aged 50–65 years carries a risk of 1 in 50000
    E. **False** – filtration reduces patient dose

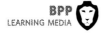

10. Which of the following will not degrade mammography image quality?
   A. Poor compression
   B. Single screen film
   C. Long exposure times
   D. Use of a boron window on the X-ray tube
   E. Moving grid

Poor compression and long exposure times can both cause image degradation through motion blur. Beryllium windows are used because of their low attenuation properties.

---

10. A. **False** – poor compression will decrease degrade image quality
   B. **True** – single screen films reduce parallax
   C. **False** – long exposure times can increase motion blur
   D. **False** – berllyium windows are used because of their low attenuation properties
   E. **True** – grids help to reduce scatter and help to maximise image quality

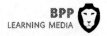

Chapter 8

Special radiographic techniques

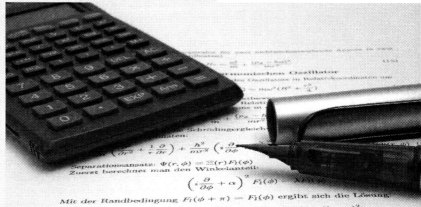

Special radiographic techniques

Please answer all questions true or false. There is no negative marking.

> 1. Advantages to high voltage radiography include
>   A. Increased patient dose
>   B. Improved patient penetration
>   C. Improved film blackening
>   D. Reduced scatter reaching the film
>   E. Improved radiographic contrast

The advantages of high voltage radiography include the following:

- Decreased patient dose
- More efficient patient penetration
- More efficient film blackening.

There are disadvantages to the use of high voltage techniques. These include reduced radiographic contrast and an increase in the amount of scatter reaching the film. To reduce the amount of scatter a grid can be used; however this has the disadvantage of causing an increase in patient dose.

1. A. **False** – patient dose is lowered
    B. **True** – penetration is improved
    C. **True** – film blackening is improved
    D. **False** – increase in forward scatter, therefore more scatter reaching the film
    E. **False** – contrast is reduced

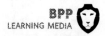

2. Macroradiography
   A. Increasing the size of the focal spot will result in an increase in the size of the penumbra (all other variables are kept constant)
   B. Focal spots of 0.3 mm or less should be aimed for
   C. The magnification ratio is equivalent to the focus-film distance minus the focus-object distance
   D. Entrance dose may be higher than in conventional radiography
   E. Mammography is a form of macroradiography

Macroradiography is magnification radiography. A good example of where the principles of macroradiography are in use is in mammography. The magnification ratio is given by the equation:

Magnification ratio = Focus-film distance / Focus-object distance

Simple geometric principles show that by increasing the size of the focal spot while keeping other variables (focus-film distance, focus-object distance and fixed object size) constant, then the penumbra will increase. This will increase the geometric unsharpness. To avoid this, the focal spot should be kept as small as possible within the rating capabilities of a tube.

Given the equation above, magnification can be achieved in several ways. One such way is to keep the focus-film distance fixed and reduce the focus-object distance ie bring the patient closer to the tube focus. This will result in increasing the entrance dose to the patient. Two important points should be recognised when this is done:

• The irradiated area should be made as small as possible to minimise dose. This can be done with effective collimation.
• An air gap will be created and this will obviate the need for a grid.

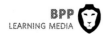

2. A. **True** – increasing the focal spot size results in a larger penumbra
    B. **True** – to minimise the geometric unsharpness caused by a large focal spot
    C. **False** – equivalent to the focus-film distance/focus-object distance
    D. **True** – the patient may be brought closer to the source, hence higher entrance dose
    E. **True** – mammography is a form of macroradiography

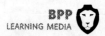

3. Regarding paediatric radiology
   A. Grids with a ratio higher than 1:8 should not be used
   B. Immobilisation may be required
   C. High-attenuation materials such as carbon fibre should be used for table tops
   D. The risk from X-rays to children is greater than in adults
   E. Additional filtration may be required

Children are at a greater risk from X-rays than adults. Therefore principles to minimise doses should be used. Some important features of paediatric radiology include:

- Exposure times should be kept as short as possible
- Added filtration may be needed. This is normally 1 mm aluminium plus 0.1–0.2 mm of copper. This is required for adequate beam hardening
- Low-attenuation materials should be used for the tabletops, cassette cases, etc
- Immobilisation may be required either from a person or from appropriate devices
- Grids are often not needed because children produce less scatter. If they are used the grid ratio should not exceed 1:8.

3. A. **True** – this will help to minimise the increased dose associated with using a grid
   B. **True** – to minimise motion blur
   C. **False** – low attenuation materials are required
   D. **True** – the risk is much greater in children compared to adults
   E. **True** – for adequate beam hardening

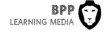

Chapter 9
Gamma imaging

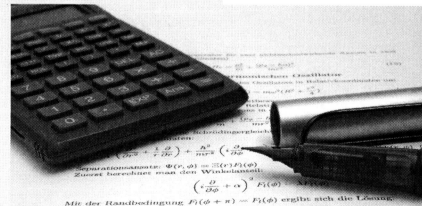

Gamma imaging

Please answer all questions true or false. There is no negative marking.

> 1. The scintillation crystal used in gamma cameras
>   A. Is normally composed of NaI
>   B. Is activated with caesium
>   C. Has a low atomic number and density
>   D. Is approximately 50 mm thick
>   E. Is hygroscopic

The scintillation crystal used in a gamma camera (also known as Anger cameras) is usually composed of thallium activated NaI. This has a relatively high atomic number which will increase the absorption probability. It is generally about 500 mm in diameter and about 10 mm thick. The crystal is very fragile and is easily damaged by temperature fluctuations. To protect it from the elements it is generally encased in an aluminium housing with one transparent face.

---

1. A. **True** – the scintillation crystal is made of NaI
    B. **False** – activated with thallium
    C. **False** – it has a high atomic number and density
    D. **False** – 10 mm thick
    E. **True** – the crystal is hygroscopic

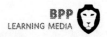

2. With regard to the scintillation crystal
   A. It converts incident light photons into electrons
   B. The thickness of the crystal has no effect on spatial resolution
   C. It is connected to photomultiplier tubes
   D. Linear defects in the image represent a crack in the crystal
   E. With a 12.5 mm NaI (Tl) crystal and 140 keV incident photons interactions in the crystal will be of the order of 90%

The scintillation crystal converts incident gamma photons into light photons. Since the gamma photons have vastly greater energy than the light photons, approximately 5000 light photons are produced for every incident gamma photon.

A photocathode is attached to the scintillation crystal and this converts the light photons to electrons. A photomultiplier tube is attached to the scintillation crystal. At 140 keV approximately 90% of incident photons undergo interactions within the crystal. The figure drops for increasing energy and/or decreasing thickness, so a thinner crystal will have decreased sensitivity. A thicker crystal will stop more incident photons but they may interact at various depths in the crystal. This results in a decreased spatial resolution. Various artefacts can occur with gamma cameras and a crack in the crystal will produce a linear defect.

2. A. **False** – it converts gamma photons into light photons
   B. **False** – thicker crystals decrease spatial resolution
   C. **True** – the photomultiplier tube is attached to the scintillation crystal
   D. **True** – cracks in the crystal result in a linear defect
   E. **True** – approximately 90% of interactions occur with this thickness and energy

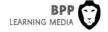

3.   The collimator of a gamma camera
   A.   Is principally used to reduce dose to the patient
   B.   Is most often made of lead
   C.   Spatial resolution is improved by increasing the size of the lead septa separating the holes
   D.   A pinhole collimator may be used when imaging the thyroid
   E.   System sensitivity and spatial resolution are inversely related

The collimator is present between the patient and the camera. The main purpose of it is to act as a funnel for the photons emitted from the patient and they provide spatial information. It does not reduce dose to the patient. They are commonly made of lead and contain many holes. Between the holes are lead septa. The spatial resolution will be increased if:

- The holes are made smaller
- The lead septa are made thicker (hence the holes made smaller)
- The collimator is made thicker.

These changes will increase the spatial resolution but will decrease the actual number of photons reaching the scintillation crystal (more will be absorbed in the collimator) and so the sensitivity will decrease. Hence sensitivity and spatial resolution are inversely related. Several different shapes of collimator exist and a pinhole collimator is often used to image small things such as the thyroid gland.

3.   A.   **False** – it does not reduce dose
   B.   **True** – often made of lead
   C.   **True** – this is one of the ways to improve spatial resolution
   D.   **True** – pinhole collimators are used when imaging smaller structures
   E.   **True** – sensitivity and spatial resolution are inversely related

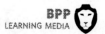

4. Which of the following can cause artefacts in nuclear medicine imaging?
   A. Cracked scintillation crystals
   B. Patient motion
   C. Metal objects on the patient can mimic pathology
   D. Incorrect setting of the pulse height analyser window
   E. Failure of a photomultiplier tube

Artefacts can occur with any imaging modality. As with other imaging modalities, movement (voluntary or involuntary) can result in motion artefacts. Cracked crystals cause linear artefacts. Metal objects **on** the patient can absorb emitted photons and can mimic a pathological cold lesion. A similar situation can occur if there is failure of a photo-multiplier tube; however this can be easily detected. Incorrectly setting the window of the pulse height analyser can result in the detection of the Compton tail instead of the photo-peak.

---

4. A. **True** – linear artefacts
   B. **True** – movement artefact
   C. **True** – pathological cold lesions
   D. **True** – detection of Compton Tail
   E. **True** – cold spot

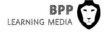

5.   The following are true regarding the pulse height spectrum
     A.   Only the pulses in the photo-peak are useful for spatial resolution
     B.   The photo-peak shows pulses that have occurred because of photoelectric interactions after initial Compton interactions in the patient
     C.   Pulse pile-up is caused by two or more photons being detected at the same time
     D.   A wider window on the pulse height analyser results in image quality improvement
     E.   The pulse pile-up peak occurs to the right of the main photo-peak

The pulse height spectrum has several components. The Compton tail occurs because gamma rays have interacted in the patient or in the scintillation crystal. The photo-peak is produced by pulses produced entirely by photoelectric interactions in the crystal without any prior Compton interactions (either in the patient, collimator or the crystal).

If two pulses are detected at the same time they can be read as one jumbo sized pulse. Hence to the right of the photo-peak a smaller pulse may occur. The photo-peak pulses are useful for spatial resolution since they have not had any prior interaction before reaching the crystal and hence should not have had any significant course deviation whilst exiting the body. Since the photo-peak is used for spatial resolution, a narrow window setting on the pulse height analyser will improve it. However, since fewer photons will be detected because of the narrower window setting there will be concomitant image quality degradation and a longer acquisition time.

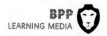

5. A. **True** – since there have been no other interactions
    B. **False** – the photo-peak shows only pulses produced by photoelectric interaction without prior Compton interaction
    C. **True** – this is the reason for the pulse pile-up peak
    D. **False** – a wider pulse height analyser will result in decreased spatial resolution
    E. **True** – the pulse pile-up peak occurs to the right

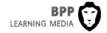

6. The following radio-nuclides are produced in a cyclotron
    A. In^{111}
    B. I^{123}
    C. Tc^{99m}
    D. Xe^{133}
    E. C^{11}

A cyclotron produces radio-nuclides by bombarding atoms with high energy protons. Cyclotron produced radio-nuclides are generally not in wide use currently. They tend to decay by beta+ decay or electron capture.

6. A. **True** – produced in a cyclotron
    B. **True** – produced in a cyclotron
    C. **False** – produced in a generator
    D. **False** – produced as product of nuclear fission
    E. **True** – produced in a cyclotron

7. Radio-pharmaceuticals
   A. Should all have very long half-lives to aid image acquisition
   B. The effective half-life can be longer than the physical half-life
   C. Should have their activity checked and recorded before being administered to the patient
   D. Manual handling should be kept to a minimum
   E. Tc^{99m} is generator-produced

Radio-pharmaceuticals are required when performing nuclear medicine investigations. Like all radioactive substances they have a half-life. The effective half-life is a combination of the physical half-life and biological half-life (this is due to the clearance of the radio-pharmaceutical from the body). The relationship is:

$$1/T_{effective} = 1/T_{biological} + 1/T_{physical}$$

This relationship means the effective half-life is **always** shorter than the biological half-life or the physical half-life. Most nuclear medicine investigations deliver an effective dose of less than 5 mSv.

To minimise the dose to patients certain precautions are undertaken. These include using isotopes with half-lives that are suitable for the investigation. They should not be too long or too short. Patients should also drink copious amounts of water in order to empty the bladder frequently. This helps to reduce the dose to the pelvic organs, gonads and pelvic bone marrow. In pregnant patients, obviously the risk-benefit ratio needs to be assessed.

According to ARSAC regulations, before administration of a radio-pharmaceutical the activity must be checked and recorded. This is done with a dose callibrator that produces an ionisation current proportional to the gamma activity. Technicians in the nuclear medicine labs are often responsible for the preparation. They must therefore take adequate protection measures. These include keeping handling to a minimum, using long handled tongs for handling if possible, leaded syringes, etc. They will also wear ring dosimeters

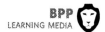

to monitor the dose received by the hand/fingers as this can be high enough for them to become classified workers.

---

7. A. **False** – the half-life should be suitable for the investigation
    B. **False** – this can never happen
    C. **True** – according ARSAC guidelines
    D. **True** – this helps keep exposure to a minimum
    E. **True** – Tc^{99m} is produced in a generator

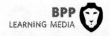

8.   Regarding the technetium generator
      A.   Mo^{99} has a half-life of 6 hours
      B.   Sterilised water is used to elute the technetium (Tc)
            when needed
      C.   The generator is replaced after 1 month
      D.   Tc^{99m} produces 140 keV gamma rays
      E.   Transient equilibrium is reached in approximately
            24 hrs

Technetium 99 m is used in about 90% of radio-nuclide investigations. It decays producing gamma rays at 140 keV. It is generator produced. The generator has a life of approximately 1 week. The parent nuclide is molybdenum^{99} that decays to Tc^{99m} by beta minus decay. The Tc^{99m} then decays by isomeric transition to Tc^{99}.

Mo^{99} → beta minus decay, T$_{1/2}$ 67 hrs → Tc^{99m} → 140 keV gamma rays, T$_{1/2}$ 6 hrs → Tc^{99}

After about 24 hrs the Tc^{99m} (daughter) and Mo^{99} (parent) are in transient equilibrium. At this point the activity of the parent and the daughter is equal and they both decay together with a half-life equal to that of the parent. It is at this point that the Tc^{99m} is eluted. Sterile saline is used as the eluting agent. Since the Mo and Tc have different chemical properties the Tc can be eluted from the generator by means of a chemical reaction. The Tc is washed off as sodium pertechnetate. This process takes several minutes and leaves the Mo^{99} behind to continue to decay and form more Tc^{99m}.

---

8.   A.   **False** – the half-life of Tc^{99m} is about 6 hours
      B.   **False** – sterile saline is used as the eluting agent
      C.   **False** – the generator has a life of about 1 week
      D.   **True** – 140 keV gamma rays are produced by Tc^{99m}
      A.   **True** – transient equilibrium is reached after 24 hrs

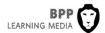

> 9. Desirable characteristics of radio-pharmaceuticals include
>   A. Emission of gamma rays with energy above 500 keV
>   B. Low specific activity
>   C. Decay to a stable daughter product
>   D. Emission of gamma rays only
>   E. Low toxicity

The desirable characteristics of a radio-nuclide include:

- A physical half-life of several hours
- No alpha or beta emission and gamma rays with energy between 50–300 keV, ideally about 150 keV and preferably mono-energetic
- Ready availability
- High specificity with low background activity
- Decay to stable daughter or one with a very long half-life
- No effect on metabolism
- Low toxicity and stable *in vivo* and *in vitro*
- Relatively inexpensive.

9. A. **False** – energy should be 50–300 keV
   B. **False** – high specific activity
   C. **True** – stable daughter product or very long life
   D. **True** – no alpha or beta emission
   E. **True** – low toxicity and stable *in vivo* and *in vitro*

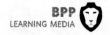

10. Concerning photo-multiplier tubes
    A. Require a photo-cathode for operation
    B. Contain a series of dynodes that act as an electronic lens
    C. Amplification is of the order of 10^6
    D. The photo-cathode produces 10 electrons per incident photon
    E. A potential difference of 1–1.2kV exists across the PMT

Photo-multiplier tubes (PMTs) consist of an evacuated glass envelope. On one side is a photocathode and on the opposite side is an anode. The photocathode emits electrons when incident photons strike it. Approximately 5–10 incident photons are required to eject 1 electron. This electron is then accelerated towards the anode via a series of dynodes.

Each dynode, when struck by an incident electron, releases more electrons. Since each dynode in the chain is at a higher potential than its predecessor the electrons not only accelerate towards the anode but also increase in number. In this manner there is considerable amplification of any signal.

There are between 10–12 dynodes in the chain and each has a potential difference of about 100 v. This results in a total potential difference across the tube of 1–1.2 kV. Each dynode releases about four electrons for every one that hits it. This results in an amplification of approximately 10^6.

---

10. A. **True** – a photo-cathode and an anode are required
    B. **False** – the dynodes act as amplifiers
    C. **True** – amplification is in the region of 10^6
    D. **False** – the photocathode produces 1 electron per 5–10 incident photon
    E. **True** – the potential difference is 1–1.2 kV across the PMT

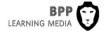
BPP
LEARNING MEDIA

11. Positron emission tomography
    A. Uses positron emitters such as Tc^{99m}
    B. Is based on the simultaneous detection of two 511 keV photons that are produced when a positron combines with an electron
    C. A ring of CsI detectors is used
    D. Generally uses generator-produced radio-nuclides
    E. Up to 20000 detectors are used for each PET scanner

Positron emission tomography (PET) uses the fact that an electron and a positron combine to annihilate each other and release energy. This reaction, which only occurs when the emitted positron has lost all its kinetic energy (ie has come to rest), causes the release of two 511 keV photons that travel in exact opposite directions. Positron emitters tend to be neutron poor and they are produced in cyclotrons. They are short-lived and include C^{11}, O^{15}, and F^{18}. Fluorine^{18} is the most commonly used.

The detectors form a ring around the patient. They are generally made of bismuth germanate and can number 10000–20000. As the two photons are released in opposite directions they can be used to calculate positional information. Scatter can obviously occur but this is minimised by using collimators between each ring of detectors.

11. A. **False** – Tc^{99m} is not a positron emitter
    B. **True** – this is the basis for PET
    C. **False** – the detectors are made of bismuth germanate
    D. **False** – positron emitters are produced in cyclotrons
    E. **True** – 10000–20000 detectors for each PET scanner

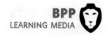

12. Regarding gamma camera quality control
    A. Field uniformity refers to the ability to produce a uniform distribution of activity
    B. Field uniformity can be tested by using a flat sealed plate of Co^{57} called a flood field
    C. Intrinsic floods are performed with the collimator
    D. Extrinsic floods are produced without the collimator
    E. Modern cameras should have a uniformity of better than 2%

The field uniformity refers to how well the gamma camera is able to reproduce a uniform field. It is checked by placing a large (larger than the field of view) flat plate that contains a radioactive source – flood field or sheet phantom. Commonly Tc^{99m} or Co^{57} are used.

Non-uniformity of greater than 10% is not acceptable for clinical imaging. In modern cameras a field uniformity of better than 2% between two adjacent areas is to be expected. Floods can be checked with and without the collimator. Extrinsic floods are checked with the collimator, and intrinsic floods without.

---

12. A. **True** – by definition
    B. **True** – a flood field or sheet phantom
    C. **False** – intrinsic floods are done without the collimator
    D. **False** – extrinsic floods are done with the collimator
    E. **True** – better than 2% should be expected

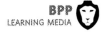

13. Regarding the effective dose
  A. Measured in Sieverts
  B. The liver has the highest tissue weighting factor of 0.12
  C. Most nuclear medicine tests have an effective dose of <5 mSv
  D. A 600MBq Tc^{99m} bone scan delivers an effective dose of approximately 5 mSv
  E. Nuclear medicine scans that aim to localise sources of infection and/or inflammation have, on average, the lowest effective doses

---

In nuclear medicine investigations the dose to a patient is not related to how many images are taken or which part of the body is being imaged. The source is internal. The excretory organs and those of interest generally receive the highest doses.

Since individual tissues and organs respond differently to radiation the tissue weighting factor for organs must be remembered when calculating effective doses. The effective dose is measured in Sieverts. The product of the absorbed organ dose and its tissue weighting factor is the effective dose to that organ. Summing for all the organs in the body will give the total effective dose.

Gallium scans used to help localise occult infections and inflammation are some of the highest dose investigations performed. They give an effective dose of approximately 20 mSv.

---

13. A. **True** – Sievert is the term used for the measurement of dose
  B. **False** – it is not the liver but the gonads that have the highest tissue weighting factor
  C. **True** – the majority of nuclear medicine tests deliver an effective dose < 5mSv
  D. **True** – approximately 5 mSv
  E. **False** – they have some of the highest effective doses

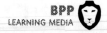

14. Concerning image noise in nuclear medicine
    A. It is the main determinant of image quality
    B. Quantum mottle plays only a minimal role in image noise
    c, Increasing the image acquisition time will decrease noise
    D. Increasing the administered dose will increase the image noise
    E. Signal-to-noise ratio is equal to N/N^2 where N is the number of absorbed photons per pixel

---

Image noise in nuclear medicine is no different to noise in other imaging modalities. It can be divided into random and structured noise. Random noise (quantum mottle) is the result of a statistical variation in the number of photons being detected. It is a major source of image noise. It is related to the number of photons by the equation $N^{\frac{1}{2}}$. The signal-to-noise ratio is represented by $N/N^{\frac{1}{2}}$. So, if the number of photons is increased then the signal-to-noise ratio will increase exponentially. With this in mind the ways one can increase the number of photons being detected include:

- Increasing the acquisition time
- Increasing the administered radioactivity to the patient.

Structured noise can include non-uniformities in the camera, overlying objects, etc. Electronic noise is another source that is caused by instability in the circuits between the receptor and viewer.

---

14. A. **True** – noise is the main determinant of image quality
    B. **False** – quantum mottle plays an important role in random noise
    C. **True** – this allows the detection of more photons
    D. **False** – this has no effect on noise in nuclear medicine
    E. **False** – equal to $N/N^{1/2}$

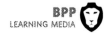

15. Concerning system resolution in nuclear medicine
    A. Scatter in the patient has no effect on image quality in nuclear medicine because the collimators will remove it
    B. It is not affected by body habitus
    C. It is of the order of 5–10 mm dependent on which collimator is used
    D. It can be tested using a line source
    E. The Full Width Half Maximum is a measure of the spatial resolution of a system

---

The ability to see two separate radioactive sources is the resolution for that particular system. To test this, a line source (a thin tube filled with radioactive material) is placed in front of the camera and a plot count is made. This graph is called the Line Spread Function. Measuring the Full Width Half Maximum (FWHM) of the Line Spread Function is often used to compare the resolutions of different systems.

Generally the resolution of gamma cameras is approximately 5–10 mm. Scatter of the photons in the patient causes this spread. Anything that will increase scatter in the patient will hence worsen the system resolution. So increased body mass will worsen the system resolution of an organ. Increasing the distance between the source and the detector will also worsen the system resolution.

---

15. A. **False** – scatter in the patient causes spread
    B. **False** – increased body mass degrades the system resolution
    C. **True** – the resolution is of the order of 5–10 mm
    D. **True** – this is how the resolution is tested
    E. **True** – it can be used to compare the spatial resolution between systems

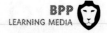

16. Regarding gamma camera collimators
    A. Converging collimators magnify the image
    B. Diverging collimators minify the image
    C. High-sensitivity collimators have fewer holes than lower-sensitivity collimators
    D. High-energy collimators have thin septa and long holes
    E. Collimators are generally made of lead

Collimators in gamma imaging are used for spatial information. Parallel hole collimators do not change the object size. Converging hole collimators magnify the image, and diverging collimators minify the image. The collimators are generally made of lead.

Collimator sensitivity and spatial resolution are generally inversely related, ie if sensitivity increases the spatial resolution decreases. Spatial resolution will increase if the holes are made smaller (thicker septa) and/or longer (the collimator is made thicker). These changes will cause fewer photons to reach the crystal and sensitivity is reduced. Therefore, high-sensitivity collimators may have larger holes and fewer of them; thinner septa; and are also themselves thinner. High-energy collimators need thicker septa to stop photons travelling through them.

16. A. **True** – converging collimators magnify
    B. **True** – diverging collimators minify
    C. **True** – higher-sensitivity collimators have fewer holes
    D. **False** – high-energy collimators require thicker septa
    E. **True** – collimators in nuclear medicine are generally made of lead

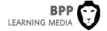

17. Regarding the pulse height analyser (PHA) in a nuclear medicine system
    A. It is found between the detector and the counting system
    B. It can be set to detect more than one photo-peak
    C. A wide window setting produces images faster
    D. A narrow window setting will cause degradation of image quality
    E. The peak is directly proportional to the energy of the gamma ray absorbed in the scintillation crystal

The pulse height analyser is a very important part of the gamma imaging circuit. It is located between the detector and the counting part of the imaging system. It is designed to select which part of the pulse height spectrum is used to form the image. Ideally you only want to detect those photons that have come from the body without any attenuation. These photons cause the photo-peak on the spectrum. Therefore, using your pulse height analyser you can tell the computer to 'read' only those photons with energy above a certain cut-off, eg 140 keV. This will effectively cause the computer not to 'see' the Compton tail of the spectrum and the pulse pile-up. The 'window' (as a percentage) determines the limits that will be detected eg 140keV +/– 10%. Using a wider window will detect more photons and hence result in quicker image formation. However, since more photons of lower and higher energies are being detected the image quality will be degraded. The pulse height analyser can be used to detect more than one photo-peak by using several window settings.

17. A. **True** – it is found between the detector and the counting system
    B. **True** – the PHA can detect more than one photopeak
    C. **True** – this will produce images faster but the image quality will be degraded
    D. **False** – a wide window will cause image degradation
    E. **True** – the peak is proportional to the incident gamma ray energy

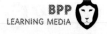

18. In a 750MBq cardiac MUGA scan using Tc^{99m}
   A. The effective dose of the procedure is approximately 6 mSv
   B. A shorter acquisition time will decrease the dose
   C. Collimators will decrease the dose
   D. Regular bladder emptying should be encouraged
   E. Changing the crystal will allow better image quality

For this procedure the effective dose is around 6 mSv. Acquisition time will have no effect on dose to the patient since the radioactive source is intrinsic to the patient. Collimators are not used to decrease dose in gamma imaging. They are used to determine spatial information.

In all nuclear medicine imaging it is advised to drink plenty and frequently void. These measures help to limit the dose to the pelvic bone marrow, organs and gonads.

Whilst collimators can be changed for different examinations the scintillation crystal cannot.

18. A. **True** – the effective dose is approximately 6mSv
   B. **False** – this has no effect on the dose
   C. **False** – collimators have no effect on the dose
   D. **True** – this is one way to minimise dose to the pelvic region
   E. **False** – the scintillation crystal cannot be changed

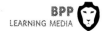

Chapter 10

Digital radiology

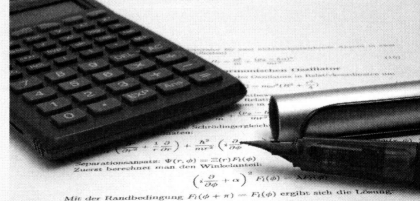

Digital radiology

Please answer all questions true or false. There is no negative marking.

---

1. Which of the statements regarding Fourier analysis are correct
    A. Fourier analysis involves breaking down an image into a series of sine waves
    B. Aliasing is most often produced by sampling at too high a frequency
    C. Aliasing is responsible for streak artefacts in computed tomography
    D. The Nyquist frequency is equal to twice the sampling frequency
    E. The modulation transfer function increases as the spatial resolution increases

---

Fourier analysis is a mathematical way in which space- or time-varying data can be transformed into a series of frequencies of sine and cosine, hence transforming an analogue signal into a pattern of frequencies. This further allows for more complex mathematical transformation used in image processing.

Aliasing occurs when digital sampling of an analogue signal is too low, causing fine detail of the original analogue signal to be lost. Aliasing is responsible for streak artefacts in CT and reverse flow artefacts seen in Doppler if the frequency of sampling is too low. To avoid aliasing, the Nyquist criterion is used which states that the sampling frequency must be twice that of the analogue frequency being sampled. The Nyquist frequency describes the maximum analogue frequency that can be accurately sampled, hence this is equal to half the sampling frequency.

The modulation transfer frequency is a measure of the ratio of output signal to input signal, hence it measures how accurately systems where signals undergo change work. In an ideal situation

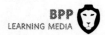

the transfer modulation frequency would be 100%, ie it would accurately transfer all available information without loss. In radiology the higher the spatial resolution the less likely a system will be able to accurately modulate information.

---

1. A. **True** – Fourier analysis involves breaking down an image into a series of sine waves
   B. **False** – aliasing is most often produced by sampling at too low a frequency
   C. **True** – aliasing is responsible for streak artefacts in computed tomography
   D. **False** – the Nyquist frequency is equal to half the sampling frequency
   E. **False** – the modulation transfer function decreases as the spatial resolution increases

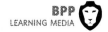

2.   Regarding the general principles of computed radiography
      A.   Computed radiography uses photostimulable phosphors such as barium fluorohalide doped with silver (BaFX:Ag)
      B.   The halide is comprised of 85% bromide and 15% iodine
      C.   The polyester base used in computed radiography is typically 3 mm thick
      D.   A computed radiography reader uses a stationary mirror
      E.   Once the computed radiography plate is read it needs to be wiped prior to re-use

Computed radiography makes use of a photostimulable phosphor. Phosphors are materials able to absorb energy and emit it again in the form of light, whether this is immediate (fluorescence) or delayed (phosphorence). Photostimulable phosphors are phosphors which emit the stored energy when exposed to light.

A commonly used photostimulable phosphor is barium flurohalide doped with europium (BaFX:Eu). The halide is a combination of bromide (85%) and iodine (15%). This is laid on a polyester base which is 0.3 mm thick to form a plate which is contained within a cassette, similar to conventional radiography. The image plate is read using a laser which is moved across the plate by reflecting off a rotating mirror. The imaging plate needs to be wiped before being used again, by exposing it to a bright light source.

2.   A.   **False** – computed radiography uses photostimulable phosphors such as barium fluorohalide doped with europium (BaFX:Eu)
      B.   **True** – the halide is comprised of 85% bromide and 15% iodine
      C.   **False** – the polyester base used in computed radiography is typically 0.3 mm thick
      D.   **False** – a computed radiography reader uses a rotating mirror
      E.   **True** – once the computed radiography plate is read it needs to be wiped prior to re-use

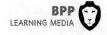

3. Regarding indirect conversion digital radiography
   A. Indirect digital radiography detectors commonly use amorphous selenium detector arrays
   B. Indirect digital radiography detectors commonly use gadolinium oxysulphide phosphors
   C. Caesium iodide crystals internally reflect light, thus reducing spread of light in the phosphor layer
   D. Caesium iodide crystals are grown perpendicular to the detector surface
   E. Gadolinium oxysulphide is used as an alternative to caesium iodide as the light spread within the phosphor is less

Digital radiography systems make use of Thin-Film Transistor (TFT) arrays, ie a grid of transistors which are able to amplify and store electrical charge. This electrical signal can be read to give a fairly instant output from the array and an image can be formed.

Digital radiography is commonly divided into two groups depending on how the X-rays are converted into an electrical charge. Indirect conversion uses a phosphor to convert X-rays to light, and then uses photodiodes within an amorphous silicon TFT array to convert the light to electrical charge.

Caesium iodide and gadolinium oxysulphide are two common phosphors used. Caesium iodide is a crystalline structure where the crystals are grown perpendicular to the detector array and the crystals are able to internally reflect the light produced in the crystals, thus reducing light spread within the phosphor and allowing for a thicker layer. Light spread within gadolinium oxysulphide is greater; however it is a rare earth material and is very efficient at converting X-rays into light so a thinner phosphor layer can be used.

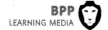

3.   A.   **False** – indirect digital radiography detectors commonly use amorphous silicon detector arrays

B.   **True** – indirect digital radiography detectors commonly use gadolinium oxysulphide phosphors

C.   **True** – caesium iodide crystals internally reflect light thus reducing spread of light in the phosphor layer

D.   **True** – caesium iodide crystals are grown perpendicular to the detector surface

E.   **False** – gadolinium oxysulphide is used as an alternative to caesium iodide as the light spread within the phosphor is greater

4. With regard to pixels and bit-depth, which of the following are correct
A. For the same number of pixels, increasing the field of view decreases the pixel size
B. Increasing the pixel size reduces the spatial resolution
C. The maximum number of greys stored in a pixel is determined by the bit-depth
D. An 8-bit pixel can store up to 512 levels of grey
E. Compression of an image will cause degradation of the image

---

The pixel size is determined by the field of view divided by the number of pixels, hence increasing the field of view increases the pixel size. As the pixel size becomes larger, each given area of the image is made up of fewer pixels so the more coarse and grainy the image becomes.

A binary system of storage of information works on storing information as sets of zero or 1. The number of bits refers to how many sets of zero or 1 can be used to store information. The bit-depth determines the number of values that can be stored in a pixel, ie a greater bit-depth results in a greater number of levels of grey. An 8-bit memory can hold 2^8 numbers = 256 possibilities. Compression can be lossless or lossy depending on the compression technique used; hence not all compression techniques will result in a loss of image quality.

---

4. A. **False** – for the same number of pixels, increasing the field of view increases the pixel size
B. **True** – increasing the pixel size reduces the spatial resolution
C. **True** – the maximum number of greys stored in a pixel is determined by the bit-depth
D. **False** – an 8-bit pixel can store up to 256 levels of grey
E. **False** – compression of an image can be lossless

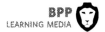

5. Which of the following statements regarding image quality in computed radiography are true
   A. Photostimulable phosphors have a wide dynamic range of about 1000:1
   B. The light intensity emitted by the photostimulable phosphor has a linear relationship with the X-ray dose
   C. A computed radiography system has greater latitude than a film-screen equivalent
   D. Computed radiography systems generally have a higher spatial resolution than film-screen equivalents
   E. Computed radiography systems generally have a higher contrast than film-screen equivalents

---

Photostimulable phosphors have a wide dynamic range of about 10000:1. Unlike the characteristic curve formed by film-screen combinations, a graph of the log of the X-ray dose against the log of the light emitted from the phosphor upon reading is linear. The range of doses that can be identified - the latitude - is much greater in computed radiography than film-screen combinations.

The initial signal obtained from computed radiography systems has to undergo processing to enhance the image and give it an appearance similar to that obtained in film-screen combinations. These techniques are used to enhance the contrast, which is generally higher than in film-screen combinations post-processing. Resolution in small computed radiography plates is generally around 5.5 lp mm^{-1} whereas film-screen combinations typically give resolutions of 8 lp mm^{-1}.

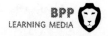

5. A. **False** – photostimulable phosphors have a wide dynamic range of about 10000:1

    B. **False** – the log of the light intensity emitted by the photostimulable phosphor has a linear relationship with the log of the X-ray dose

    C. **True** – a computed radiography system has greater latitude than a film-screen equivalent

    D. **False** – computed radiography systems generally have a lower spatial resolution than film-screen equivalents

    E. **True** – computed radiography systems generally have a higher contrast than film-screen equivalents

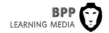

6.   Regarding PACS and DICOM
      A.   PACS is an acronym for Picture Archiving Computer
           System
      B.   PACS provides the ability to view images
           instantaneously on different monitors
      C.   If the computer display meets DICOM standard this
           ensures adequate conditions for reporting
      D.   DICOM is an acronym for Digital Imaging and
           Communications in Medicine Services
      E.   Hospital monitors which display PACS images must
           meet DICOM standards

Picture Archiving and Communication Systems (PACS) are now in common use in many hospitals. A PACS is a computer system which allows the storage and visualisation of radiography images throughout a hospital, elimination of film stores and often integration with image reports and other digital patient records.

Different computers have the potential to display images differently and so computer displays are calibrated to DICOM (Digital Imaging and Communications in Medicine Services) standards. This must apply to those computer screens from which a report of the images is to be made (eg in reporting rooms) however not all displays on which the images can be viewed may meet these standards and as such carry risks when interpreting from them. Even if a hospital monitor meets DICOM standards other factors in the room such as ambient light must be taken into account when reporting from images.

6.   A.   **False** – PACS is an acronym for Picture Archiving and
                Communication Systems
      B.   **True** – PACS provides the ability to view images
                instantaneously on different monitors
      C.   **False** – other factors must also be taken into
                consideration
      D.   **True** – DICOM is an acronym for Digital Imaging and
                Communications in Medicine Services
      E.   **False** – hospital monitors which display PACS images
                must meet DICOM standards if a report is to be
                made from them

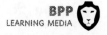

7. Which of the following statements regarding direct conversion digital radiography are true?
   A. Direct digital radiography uses an amorphous silicon TFT array
   B. Gadolinium oxysulphide may be used as a phosphor in direct conversion systems
   C. The upper electrode is connected to a high-voltage negative potential
   D. The detector quantum efficiency of a digital radiography system is greater than 80%
   E. Digital radiography systems are normally more expensive than the equivalent computed radiography systems

Direct conversion digital radiography systems do not use a phosphor. Instead they use an amorphous selenium photoconductor which converts X-rays directly into electrical charge. This is placed on top of an amorphous silicon TFT array. A constant positive charge is applied to the upper surface of the amorphous selenium hence drawing the negative charge towards the upper electrode and the positive charge towards TFT array.

The detector quantum efficiency describes the efficiency of X-ray photon detection and signal production. This is reduced by noise and X-ray absorption within the systems. Digital radiography has a detector quantum efficiency of 65% compared to computed radiography and films screens which have a detector quantum efficiency of 30%.

7. A. **True** – direct digital radiography uses an amorphous silicon TFT array
   B. **False** – phosphors are not used in direct conversion systems
   C. **True** – the upper electrode is connected to a high voltage negative potential POSITIVE .
   D. **False** – the detector quantum efficiency of a digital radiography system is around 65%
   E. **True** – digital radiography systems are normally more expensive than the equivalent computed radiography systems

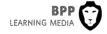

Chapter 11

Computed tomography

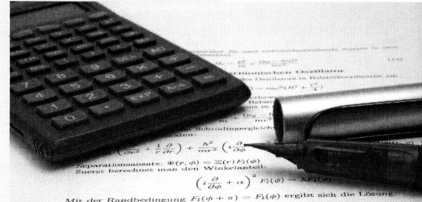

Computed tomography

Please answer all questions true or false. There is no negative marking.

> 1. With regard to the CT number
>   A. The CT number represents the median linear attenuation coefficient of tissues within the voxel
>   B. Water has a CT number of −1000
>   C. Fat has a CT number of −300
>   D. Bone has a CT number of 1500
>   E. Muscle has a CT number of 120

The CT number represents the average linear attenuation coefficient of tissues within a voxel.

$$CTn = 100 \times \frac{\mu t - \mu w}{\mu w}$$

where μw = linear attenuation coefficient of water and μt = linear coefficient of tissue within the voxel.

By definition, water therefore has a CT number of zero, whilst air (having very little density) has a CT number of −1000. Fat has a CT number in the range of −60 to −150, lung −300 to −800, muscle 40–60 and bone 500–1500.

---

1. A. **False** – the CT number represents the average linear attenuation coefficient of tissues within the voxel
    B. **False** – water has a CT number of 0
    C. **False** – fat has a CT number of −60 to −150
    D. **True** – bone has a CT number of up to 1500
    E. **False** – muscle has a CT number of 40–60

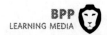

2. Which of the following statements regarding different CT scanner generations are correctly paired?
   A. First generation scanners are often referred to as a rotate-translate scanner
   B. Second generation scanners are often referred to as a rotate-translate scanner
   C. Third generation scanners are often referred to as a rotate-stationary scanner
   D. Fourth generation scanners are often referred to as a rotate-rotate scanner
   E. Fourth generation scanners are the most popular scanners in current use

First and second generation scanners are often referred to as rotate-translate scanners. The first generation had a single X-ray output source and detector which were moved through a single plane (translate) and then both source and detector were rotated 1 degree and the process repeated.

Second generation scanners used the same technology but increased the number of detectors reducing the scan time.

Third generation scanners made use of a fully rotating gantry with both the X-ray source and detector able to rotate 360 degrees around the patient and gather information (rotate-rotate).

Fourth generation scanners used a rotating source with a fixed complete ring of detectors which were stationary (rotate-stationary). This helped in reconstruction, and allowed more accurate calibration; however as the X-ray source rotated within the ring of detectors, the distance between the source and the patient was less and the dose increased significantly.

Fifth generation scanners involve different technology using an electron beam to produce X-rays (electron beam scanner). Third generation scanners are now the most widely used with large multislice scanners and improved reconstruction algorithms decreasing the scan time.

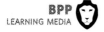

2. A. **True** – first generation scanners are often referred to as a rotate-translate scanner
    B. **True** – second generation scanners are often referred to as a rotate-translate scanner
    C. **False** – third generation scanners are often referred to as a rotate-rotate scanner
    D. **False** – fourth generation scanners are often referred to as a rotate-stationary scanner
    E. **False** – third generation scanners are the most popular scanners in current use

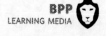

3. Regarding CT artefacts
   A. Partial volume artefact causes a small high-contrast object to appear larger than it actually is
   B. Partial volume effect is reduced when the slice thickness is increased
   C. Cone beam effect is increased with increasing numbers of slices in a multislice scanner
   D. Cone beam effect occurs due to the convergent nature of an X-ray beam
   E. High attenuation objects cause streak artefacts on CT

Partial volume effect occurs when a high-contrast object partially fills a voxel. As the CT number represents an average linear coefficient of the voxel as a whole, the high-contrast object may appear larger than its actual size. The larger the voxel size the more likely this is to happen, hence the partial volume effect is reduced when decreasing the slice thickness. Cone beam effect occurs as reconstruction algorithms assume that X-ray beams are non-divergent. Of course, X-ray beams do diverge and this effect on reconstruction algorithms becomes more pronounced with the greater number of slices, and so the reconstruction becomes more complicated. High attenuation objects such as metal cause streak artefacts, which appear as black and white lines arising from the objects.

3. A. **True** – partial volume artefact causes a small high-contrast object to appear larger than it actually is
   B. **False** – partial volume effect is reduced when the slice thickness is decreased
   C. **True** – cone beam effect is increased with increasing numbers of slices in a multislice scanner
   D. **False** – cone beam effect occurs due an X-ray beam being divergent
   E. **True** – high attenuation objects cause streak artefacts on CT

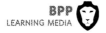

4. Regarding the pitch of CT scanners
   A. In a CT scanner, pitch is the ratio of table movement during one full rotation to slice thickness
   B. If the table moves 10 mm per rotation and the slice thickness is 5 mm, the pitch is 0.5
   C. The greater the pitch, the greater the patient dose
   D. A pitch of greater than 2 generally gives an unacceptable dose
   E. Increasing pitch results in a reduction of slice misregistration

Helical scanning techniques meant the entire gantry could be continuously rotated around the patient. Pitch is defined as the tabletop movement per rotation divided by the slice thickness, and determines how widely spaced is the helical path the gantry makes rotating around the patient. Hence if the table moves 10 mm per rotation, and the slice thickness is 5 mm, the pitch is 2. A pitch of 1 would imply the helical path covering the body with no spaces; the higher the number the more spaces and the greater the interpolation of data needed. The higher the pitch, the smaller the dose to the patient and the faster the scan time, in turn reducing slice misregistration of areas like the lung which occur due to movement artefact. In general a pitch above 2 is considered to give an unacceptable image quality.

4. A. **True** – in a CT scanner, pitch is the ratio of table movement during one full rotation to slice thickness
   B. **False** – if the table moves 10 mm per rotation and the slice thickness is 5 mm the pitch is 2
   C. **False** – the greater the pitch the less the patient dose
   D. **False** – a pitch of greater than 2 generally gives an unacceptable image quality
   E. **True** – increasing pitch results in a reduction of slice misregistration

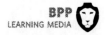

5.　Regarding CT artefacts
  A.　Motion artefacts are reduced by faster scanning times
  B.　Photon starvation often occurs between two artificial hips
  C.　Beam hardening causes streak artefacts
  D.　Ring artefacts occur due to a faulty X-ray production tube
  E.　Cupping artefact may be corrected using bow tie filters

Motion artefacts are caused by moving objects causing streak artefacts such as cardiac or lung movements. Faster scanning times have reduced the incidence of these artefacts. Photon starvation occurs when X-ray photons are attenuated by a high density object. This is most commonly seen in between two artificial hips, causing streak artefacts in the pelvis.

As an X-ray beam passes through a body it becomes progressively more attenuated hence becomes hardened. This leads to lower CT numbers in the centre of the patient than the outside. This artefact is known as beam hardening and cupping. It is corrected by both algorithms and bow-tie filters. Ring artefacts occur when a CT detector malfunctions. As the gantry rotates around the patient, each CT detector malfunction traces out a ring around the patient.

5.　A.　**True** – motion artefacts are reduced by faster scanning times
  B.　**True** – photon starvation often occurs between two artificial hips
  C.　**False** – high attenuation objects cause streak artefacts
  D.　**False** – ring artefacts occur due to a faulty X-ray detector
  E.　**True** – cupping artefact may be corrected with bow tie filters

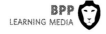

6. Which of the following statements regarding detectors in CT scanners are correct?
   A. An ideal detector in a CT machine would have a long afterglow
   B. Ionisation chambers use xenon gas at high pressure
   C. Ionisation chambers are the most common detector in multislice scanners
   D. Solid state detectors use rare earth materials such as bismuth germinate
   E. Ionisation chambers have higher detection efficiency than solid state detectors

---

An ideal detector in a CT machine would be as small as possible (to increase spatial resolution), to have a high detection efficiency, to have a wide dynamic range, and to have a small afterglow (hence to decrease scanning times).

Ionisation chambers used to be the commonest form of detector in CT. These were elongated chambers filled with xenon gas at high pressure. In multislice scanners these have been superseded by solid state detectors that use scintillants such as bismuth germinate, cadmium tungstate or rare earth materials. The detection efficiency of ionisation chambers is 60% compared to a detection efficiency of 80% for solid state detectors.

---

6. A. **False** – an ideal detector in a CT machine would have a small afterglow
   B. **True** – ionisation chambers use xenon gas at high pressure
   C. **False** – solid state chambers are the most common detector in multislice scanners
   D. **True** – solid state detectors use rare earth materials such as bismuth germinate
   E. **False** – ionisation chambers have lower detection efficiency than solid-state detectors

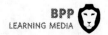

Chapter 12

Radiation detectors

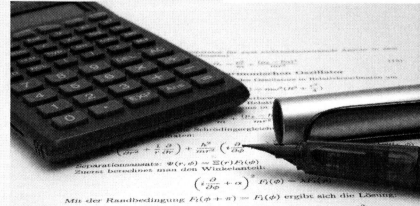

Radiation detectors

Please answer all questions true or false. There is no negative marking.

---

1. Thermo-luminescent detectors
    A. Use electron traps
    B. Produce visible light when they interact with radiation
    C. Can measure radiation doses up to 100 Gy
    D. Have a low dynamic range
    E. Demonstrate a linear response over their operating range

---

Thermo-luminescent detectors (TLDs) use electron traps to store some of the energy of an absorbed X-ray beam. On heating, the electrons are released and they produce light. The light output is proportional to the exposure. Over their operating range they show a linear response. They also have a high dynamic range of approximately 0.01 mGy to 10 Gy. They can be used for personnel dosimetry and are often used by radio-pharmacists (ring dosimeters).

---

1. A. **True** – they use electron traps to store energy
    B. **False** – they produce light when heated
    C. **False** – they can measure radiation up to 10Gy
    D. **False** – they have a high dynamic range
    E. **True** – over their operating range they show a linear response

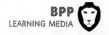

2. With regard to thermoluminescent dosimeters (TLDs)
   A. The excited electrons are trapped in the forbidden energy band
   B. They release visible light when heated to approximately 300–400°C
   C. They are commonly made from lithium fluoride
   D. They are very cheap
   E. They do not require annealing after use

Solids can be thought of as having a band structure. Three bands exist in solids and these determine some of their qualities:

- Conduction band
- Forbidden band
- Valence band.

Electron traps exist in forbidden bands, and the electrons need energy (from heat) to escape the traps. Light is produced in this process. The temperature required for this is approximately 300–400°C. After the read-out process TLDs must be carefully annealed to ensure that the same number of energy traps are available, otherwise the sensitivity of the TLD will change. This will then alter the calibration factor of the TLD.

TLDs are commonly made of lithium fluoride (LiF) since its atomic number is relatively close to that of soft tissue (Z = 8.3). They are very expensive.

---

2. A. **True** – the electron traps are in the forbidden zone
   B. **True** – the temperature required is 300–400°C
   C. **True** – they are commonly made from lithium fluoride
   D. **False** – they are very expensive
   E. **False** – they do require annealing after use

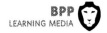

3. In comparison to a TLD, a film badge
    A. Exhibits a linear response
    B. Is relatively cheap
    C. Has a much longer time of use
    D. Is not sensitive to temperature and humidity
    E. Provides a permanent visual record

Film badges are commonly used by medical staff to monitor exposure. They differ in many qualities compared with TLDs. Some of the differences include:

- Film badges are relatively cheap compared to TLDs
- They provide a permanent record
- They are sensitive to temperature and humidity
- They can indicate the type of radiation exposure (TLDs cannot do this).

TLDs have some advantages over film badges and these include:

- They have a higher range of dose exposure over which they are useful
- They can be used for longer
- They exhibit a linear response
- They are not sensitive to humidity and ambient temperature.

---

3. A. **False** – TLDs exhibit a linear response over their operating range
    B. **True** – a film badge is relatively cheap
    C. **False** – TLDs have a longer life
    D. **False** – film badges are sensitive to both heat and humidity
    E. **True** – they can provide a permanent record

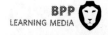

4. Concerning film badges
    A. They often contain three filters
    B. They can be used to estimate the energy of the radiation to which they have been exposed
    C. They are the most common method employed in the NHS for monitoring exposures
    D. They can indicate what type of radiation they were exposed to
    E. They have a range of usefulness of approximately 0.2 mGy – 6 Gy

---

Film badges are the most commonly used way to monitor exposure. They consist of a small case with a piece of film placed between filters. The filters allow an assessment of the penetrating power of the radiation, and hence the energy of the radiation to be estimated. They can also be used to provide information on the type of radiation exposure. Film badges do not show a linear response to exposures (unlike TLDs) and the average photon energy they were exposed to is calculated by measuring the optical density of the film. Since film can be affected by heat and temperatures, so too can film badges. They have an operating range of approximately 0.2 mGy to 6 Gy.

---

4. A. **True** – three filters are common
    B. **True** – the filters allow the energy of the radiation to be assessed
    C. **True** – they are commonly used
    D. **True** – they can provide information on the type of radiation exposure
    E. **True** – the operating range is 0.2 mGy – 6 Gy

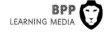

> 5. Which of the following are used to measure dose to patients and/or medical personnel?
>   A. TLDs
>   B. Film badges
>   C. Geiger counters
>   D. Ionisation chambers
>   E. Pocket ionisation chambers

All the above can be used in the measurement of dose to patients and medical personnel except Geiger counters. These are too sensitive to be used and are designed to detect low levels of radiation, eg contamination from a spill in the nuclear medicine laboratory.

---

5. A. **True** – TLDs are used
    B. **True** – film badges are commonly used
    C. **False** – Geiger counters are not used to measure dose to patients or medical personnel
    D. **True** – ionisation chambers are used
    E. **True** – pocket ionisation chambers are used

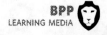

6. Regarding Geiger counters
   A. They are ionisation chambers with low voltages applied across the chamber
   B. They are too sensitive to measure diagnostic beams
   C. The true count is always higher than the measured count because of the dead time
   D. They can be used as a radiation monitor
   E. A typical dead time is approximately 300 microseconds

Geiger counters are ionisation chambers with high voltages across the chamber. They typically have a voltage difference of 300–400 V. They are very sensitive at detecting radiation – too sensitive, in fact, for diagnostic radiology. However, there is no proportionality between the count rate and the number of ionisations with GM tubes so they cannot be used as radiation monitors.

After the detection of a high energy photon a quenching agent is released to reset the Geiger counter. During this time no further ionisations can be detected. This is the 'dead time'. Typically it lasts about 300 microseconds. Because of the dead time, the true count is always higher than the measured count.

6. A. **False** – a high voltage is applied across the chamber
   B. **True** – they are too sensitive for diagnostic radiology use
   C. **True** – the true count is always higher than the measured count
   D. **False** – they can be used for radiation detection but not monitoring
   E. **True** – the typical dead time is 300 microseconds

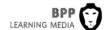

> 7. Geiger-Müller counters have the following characteristics
>   A. A central wire anode
>   B. A steel envelope
>   C. Alcohol gas is used to promote continuous discharge and improve the detection sensitivity
>   D. A thin mica window to allow the transmission of alpha particles
>   E. A thin layer of graphite inside the envelope

Geiger-Müller tubes have a central wire anode inside an envelope. The envelope is often made of glass. Inside the envelope is a thin layer of a conducting material such as graphite or silver. This is the cathode and the central wire is the anode. At one end there may be a thin mica window to allow the transmission of beta particles.

When a high energy photon enters the GM tube it initiates a photo-ionisation. This results in the production of free electrons. The electrons gain energy (because of the large potential difference between the anode and the cathode) and then cause the release of yet more electrons from the argon gas that is inside the GM tube. This process continues and causes an Electron Avalanche – a large amplification of the charge released by the incident electron. This massive output is registered as a 'click'.

In order to detect another pulse the continuous discharge from an initial pulse must be stopped. This is done by adding a quenching agent to the argon. This quenching gas is often alcohol or bromine.

7. A. **True** – the central wire acts as the anode
    B. **False** – the envelope is often made of glass
    C. **False** – alcohol gas is used as a quenching agent
    D. **False** – the mica window allows passage of beta particles
    E. **True** – there is a thin layer of graphite inside the envelope

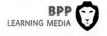

8. Ionisation chambers
   A. Can be used as photo-timers in automatic exposure control units
   B. A Geiger-Müller tube is a high-voltage ionisation chamber
   C. They require a very stable voltage supply
   D. A free air ionisation chamber has the advantage that air has a similar mean atomic number as soft tissue
   E. The reading from a free air ionisation chamber is subject to changes in pressure

An ionisation chamber consists of two plates (a cathode and an anode) with a potential difference applied across them. The free air ionisation chamber contains air between the plates. The incident photons cause ionisation of the air. The ions produced by this interaction are then attracted to either the anode or the cathode where they are detected and counted. The potential difference across the chamber needs to be high enough to collect all the liberated ions. It should not be high enough to cause amplification (like in GM tubes). However, they do not need very stable voltage supplies to operate.

They can be used to measure X-ray tube output and as accurate dosimetry devices. Free air ionisation chambers have an atomic number close to soft tissue, so the number of ionisations in air would be similar to that in an equivalent mass of soft tissue.

Exposure is calculated as follows:

Exposure = Total charge liberated / Mass of air in chamber

$E = Q / M$

Exposure has the SI units Coulombs/Kg (Roentgen is the old unit of radiation exposure).

Since the number of ionisations is dependent on the number of interactions a photon has with air molecules in the chamber, changes

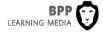

in pressure and temperature can affect the reading. Increasing the pressure will result in increased air density, increased number of interactions and hence an artificially high reading. Therefore, the ionisation chambers must be adequately calibrated.

---

8.   A.   **True** – they can be used as photo-timers
     B.   **True** – a Geiger-Müller tube is a type of ionisation chamber
     C.   **False** – they do not require a very stable power supply
     D.   **True** – air and soft tissue have similar mean atomic numbers
     E.   **True** – the reading is temperature and pressure dependent

9. The advantages scintillation crystals have when used as monitors compared to other methods include_
   A. They have a rapid response time
   B. Different scintillation crystals can be made dependent on the type of radiation that needs to be detected
   C. They have a high efficiency for detecting photons
   D. They produce an easily visible light signal that can be viewed without the need for amplification
   E. Scintillation crystals require careful annealing after use

Scintillation crystals can be used as radiation monitors. They demonstrate several advantages over other methods for radiation monitoring. These include:

- High detector efficiency
- Rapid response time
- They can be made to detect different types of radiation and/ or varying energies.

The light they produce needs amplification. This is done via photo-multiplier tubes (PMT). The same method is used in nuclear medicine.

9. A. **True** – they have a rapid response time
   B. **True** – they can be tailored to the type of radiation and/ or energy
   C. **True** – they have high detector efficiency
   D. **False** – they do require amplification
   E. **False** – TLDs require annealing after use

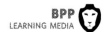

10. Pocket ionisation chambers
  A. Are mechanically sturdy
  B. Have a typical range of 0–2 mGy
  C. Cannot provide immediate readings
  D. Are easily transportable but can only be used once
  E. Can make a 'click' to signify exposure to radiation

Pocket ionisation chambers are shaped like large pens or sometimes 'bleepers'. Ionisation in the chamber causes the discharge of a charged capacitor. This can produce an immediate reading either visual or auditory – a 'click' or 'bleep' with an increasing frequency dependent on the level of exposure. They are small enough to be carried but they are fragile. They can be re-used and recharged, but they are not very accurate. A typical range is 0–2 mGy.

---

10. A. **False** – they are not very sturdy
  B. **True** – this is a typical range
  C. **False** – they can be used to provide immediate readings
  D. **False** – they can be re-used
  E. **True** – they can make either an auditory or visual reading

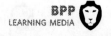

Chapter 13

Radiation hazards and protection

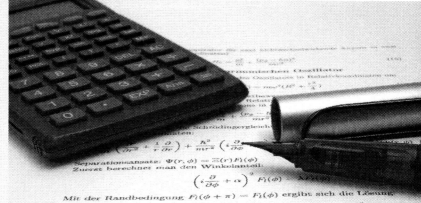

Radiation hazards and protection

Please answer all questions true or false. There is no negative marking.

---

1. Regarding radiation units
   A. Equivalent dose is measured in Jkg^{-1}
   B. Effective dose is derived from the absorbed dose multiplied by the radiation weighting factor
   C. Dose limits are given in terms of grays
   D. Effective dose is measured in sieverts
   E. Dose area product meters are measured in Gy/cm^2

Absorbed dose is the energy deposited per unit mass due to ionising radiation, and is normally measured in Jkg^{-1} but given the unit grays (Gy). 1 Jkg^{-1} is equal to 1 Gy.

Equivalent dose takes into account the relative amounts of different types of radiation needed to reach the same biological end point. For example, the relative biological effectiveness of alpha particles is much higher than gamma rays. Equivalent dose is derived by multiplying the absorbed dose by the weighting factor for the type of radiation used. Equivalent dose is also measured in Jkg^{-1} but given the unit Sievert (Sv) to distinguish it from the absorbed dose.

Effective dose takes into account the relative radiosensitivities of different tissues. Effective doses are again quoted in the Sievert unit. Dose limits apply to all types of radiation, and therefore must be given as the equivalent dose in Sieverts. Dose area product is a different way to measure patient dose. As the name suggests this is calculated as the product of the dose and beam area hence its units are Gycm^2.

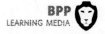

1.   A. **True** – equivalent dose is measured in Jkg^{-1}
      B. **False** – equivalent dose is derived from the absorbed dose multiplied by the radiation weighting factor
      C. **False** – dose limits are given in terms of Sieverts
      D. **True** – effective dose is measured in Sieverts
      E. **False** – dose area product meters are measured in Gycm^2

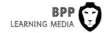

2. With regard to absorbed doses
   A. A typical absorbed dose for a PA chest film is 0.015 mGy
   B. A typical absorbed dose for 3 minutes of fluoroscopy screening can be up to 150 mGy
   C. Absorbed doses are normally lower than effective doses
   D. The typical absorbed foetal dose of a barium enema in a pregnant patient is higher than the typical absorbed adult dose of AP abdomen
   E. The typical absorbed dose of a lateral lumbar spine is 12 mGy

---

A typical absorbed dose for a PA chest is 0.15 mGy, AP abdomen is 5 mGy and lateral lumbar spine is 12 mGy. 0.015 mSv is the typical effective dose of a PA chest film. The typical absorbed foetal dose of a barium enema in a pregnant patient is 5 mGy, whilst the typical absorbed foetal dose of a CT pelvis is 10–30 mGy. Normal fluoroscopy dose rates are in the region of 5–50 mGy min^{-1}. An effective dose is usually lower than the absorbed dose.

---

2. A. **False** – a typical absorbed dose for a PA chest film is 0.15 mGy
   B. **True** – a typical absorbed dose for 3 minutes of fluoroscopy screening can be up to 150 mGy
   C. **False** – absorbed doses are normally higher than effective doses
   D. **False** – the typical absorbed foetal dose of a barium enema in a pregnant patient is the same as the typical absorbed adult dose of AP abdomen
   E. **True** – the typical absorbed dose of a lateral lumbar spine is 12 mGy

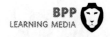

3. Regarding radiation weighting factors
    A. The radiation weighting factor of alpha particles is 20
    B. The radiation weighting factor of gamma particles is 5
    C. For the same initial energy, a particle with a higher weighting factor travels further
    D. The weighting factor for neutrons is dependent on their energy
    E. A weighting factor of 20 means that 20 times more ionisation occurs than with a weighting factor of 1

The weighting factor describes the relative biological effectiveness of different types of ionising radiation. The higher the weighting factor, the shorter a distance the particle travels as its energy is transferred, hence the more ionisation will occur in a given tissue. It should be noted that weighting factors are determined by biological endpoints, not the level of ionisation. The weighting factor of gamma particles, X-rays, electrons and beta particles is 1. Neutrons have a weighting factor of 5, 10 or 15 depending on their energy. Alpha particles have a weighting factor of 20.

---

3. A. **True** – the radiation weighting factor of alpha particles is 20
    B. **False** – the radiation weighting factor of gamma particles is 1
    C. **False** – for the same initial energy a particle with a lower weighting factor travels further
    D. **True** – the weighting factor for neutrons is dependent on their energy
    E. **False** – the weighting factor for neutrons is dependent on the relative biological effectiveness

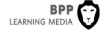

4.   With regard to the population dose
   A.   Radon on average provides the highest source of radiation exposure in the UK
   B.   Cosmic gamma rays on average provide the second highest source of natural radiation exposure
   C.   The average dose from all natural sources is roughly 3 times higher in Cornwall than across the UK in general
   D.   A 12-hour trip to Tokyo provides roughly the same absorbed dose of radiation as a PA chest film
   E.   Fallout from nuclear weapon tests contributes a higher proportion of radiation to the public than medical exposure

---

Radiation exposure to the population can be divided into natural and artificial sources.

Natural sources can be divided into one of four main groups. Radon is a radioactive inert gas that causes the largest natural source of radiation exposure. Radon on average provides an exposure of 1.3 mSv per year in the UK although this is highly variable depending on local geography. Terrestrial gamma rays provide the next highest natural source of radiation of 350 µSv per year. Cosmic gamma rays arise from sources in space and on average provide 320 µSv year^{-1} at sea level rising with increasing altitude. An approximate dose for flying at high altitude is 4 µSv hr^{-1}, so this is equivalent to 0.048 mSv for 12 hours. In comparison a typical absorbed dose for a PA chest film is 0.15 mSv. Internal radiation is produced from within the human body due to eating food and contributes 270 µSv year^{-1}. The average dose from all natural sources is roughly 2.2 mSv year^{-1}, whilst in Cornwall this may rise to 7 mSv due to a greater abundance of radon.

The largest artificial source of radiation is medical exposures with the average UK dose being 370 µSv year^{-1}, with CT imaging contributing the largest proportion of that dose. Other artificial sources of radiation are much smaller, for example the average UK dose from nuclear weapon fallout is 4 µSv year^{-1}, smoke detectors

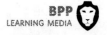

cause 0.1 μSv year^{-1} and occupational exposure causes an average of 6 μSv year^{-1}.

4.   A.   **True** – radon on average provides the highest source of radiation exposure in the UK

      B.   **True** – cosmic gamma rays on average provide the second highest source of natural radiation exposure

      C.   **True** – the average dose from all natural sources is roughly 3 times higher in Cornwall than across the UK in general

      D.   **False** – a 12-hour trip to Tokyo provides a much lower absorbed dose of radiation compared to a PA chest film.

      E.   **False** – fallout from nuclear weapon tests contributes a lower proportion of radiation to the public than medical exposure

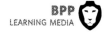

5. With regard to the differences between deterministic and stochastic effects
   A. Ulceration of the skin is a stochastic effect
   B. Once the threshold dose for a stochastic event occurs, increasing the dose does not alter the severity
   C. Sterility is a deterministic effect
   D. Most stochastic effects have repair mechanisms, an exception being cataract development of the lens
   E. Neoplasia is a deterministic effect

The effects of ionising radiation can be broadly divided into two groups, deterministic and stochastic effects. Deterministic effects have a threshold below which it is unlikely the effect will occur. Once this threshold dose is reached the chance of the effect occurring increases dramatically. Skin ulceration, sterility, erythema, hair loss, and cataracts are all deterministic effects. Most deterministic effects occur to tissues that have repair mechanisms hence the chance of the effect being caused is also dependent on the rate of radiation exposure. Cataract development is an exception to this, as the lens cannot heal itself from radiation exposure. Stochastic effects do not have threshold doses. As the radiation dose increases the risk of a stochastic effect increases, although the severity does not necessarily increase. All radiation-induced cancer is an example of a stochastic effect.

---

5. A. **False** – ulceration of the skin is a deterministic effect
   B. **False** – stochastic effects do not have a threshold dose
   C. **True** – sterility is a deterministic effect
   D. **False** – most deterministic effects have repair mechanisms except cataract development of the lens
   E. **False** – neoplasia is a stochastic effect

 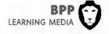

6. Which of the following are true regarding tissue weighting factors?
    A. The stomach, colon, lung, and oesophagus all have the same weighting factor
    B. The liver, stomach, and breast have a higher weighting factor than bone surface
    C. The gonads have the highest weighting factor
    D. Skin has a lower weighing factor than bone surface
    E. Weighting factors give an estimate of incidence of cancers per mSv to that organ or tissue

---

Tissue weighting factors are an indication of the radiosensitivity of various tissues and are used to calculate effective doses. They are derived from a study of survivors of the atomic weapons used in Japan in 1945. This analysed mortality from cancers, hence non-fatal cancers were not included, so they only give an estimate of mortality from a cancer rather than actually developing a cancer. For this reason the weighting factor for the thyroid is much less than would be expected as overall mortality from thyroid cancers is low. The stomach, colon, lung, and bone marrow all have a weighting factor of 0.12. The oesophagus, liver, bladder, thyroid and breast have a weighting factor of 0.05. Skin and bone surface have a weighting factor of 0.01. The gonads have weighting factor of 0.2

---

6. A. **False** – the stomach, colon and lung all have a different weighting factor from the oesophagus
    B. **True** – the liver, stomach, and breast have a higher weighting factor than bone surface
    C. **True** – the gonads have the highest weighting factor
    D. **False** – skin and bone surface have the same weighing factor
    E. **False** – weighting factors give an estimate of mortality from cancers per mSv to that organ or tissue

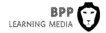

> 7. Which of the following threshold doses for deterministic effects are true?
>   A. The threshold dose for skin erythema is 2–5 Gy
>   B. The threshold dose for thyroid cancer is 25 Gy
>   C. The threshold dose for hair loss is the same as the threshold dose for skin erythema
>   D. The threshold dose for cataracts is 15 Gy
>   E. The threshold dose for fetal abnormality is higher than the threshold dose for sterility

Threshold doses apply to deterministic effects where once the radiation exceeds this level the risk of an effect occurring increases dramatically. Both skin erythema and sterility have a threshold dose of 2–5 Gy. The threshold dose for sterility is 2–3 Gy whilst the range of threshold doses for a foetal abnormality is much lower at 0.1 – 0.5 Gy, with most potential for damage in the third to eighth week. Cataracts occur above a threshold of 5 Gy. The risk of cancer developing is a stochastic effect hence threshold doses do not apply.

7.　A. **True** – the threshold dose for skin erythema is 2–5 Gy
　　B. **False** – thyroid cancer is a stochastic effect
　　C. **True** – the threshold dose for hair loss is the same as the threshold dose for skin erythema
　　D. **False** – the threshold dose for cataracts is 5 Gy
　　E. **False** – the threshold dose for foetal abnormality is lower than the threshold dose for sterility

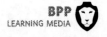

8. Regarding annual dose limits
   A. The annual effective dose limit for a member of the public is 3 mSv
   B. The annual equivalent dose limit for the lens of the eye for an employee is 5 mSv
   C. The annual equivalent dose limit for the extremities (eg skin, hands, feet) for a radiology receptionist is 50 mSv
   D. The annual equivalent dose limit for the abdomen of a female employee of reproductive age is 13 mSv
   E. The annual equivalent dose limit for the lens of the eye for a 17-year-old employee is 45 mSv

The annual effective dose for a member of the public is 1 mSv, and for an employee is 20 mSv. The equivalent dose limit for the lens of an eye in an employee is 150 mSv and 15 mSv for the public. The threshold dose for cataracts of the lens developing is 5 Gy. The equivalent dose for the extremities is 500 mSv in an employee and 50 mSv in a member of the public. Whilst the receptionist is an employee, they are not an employee who would be expected to work with ionising radiation and hence their limits are those of a member of the public. The equivalent dose limit for the abdomen of a woman of reproductive age is 13 mSv in a 3 month period, not a year. If confirmed to be pregnant, once she informs her employer the limit is adjusted to 1 mSv throughout the rest of the pregnancy. Limits for employees between 16-18 are set at $\frac{1}{3}$ the normal adult limit, hence equivalent limits of 45 mSv year^{-1} for lens of eye, 150 mSv year^{-1} for extremities, and 6 mSv effective annual dose.

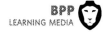

8.   A.   **False** – the annual effective dose limit for a member for the public is 1 mSv

B.   **False** – the annual equivalent dose limit for the lens of the eye for an employee is 150 mSv

C.   **True** – the annual equivalent dose limit for the extremities (eg skin, hands, feet) for a radiology receptionist is 50 mSv

D.   **False** – the equivalent dose limit for the abdomen of a female employee of reproductive age is 13 mSv in a 3-month period

E.   **True** – the annual equivalent dose limit for the lens of the eye for a 17-year-old employee is 45 mSv

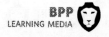

9. Which of the following regarding radiation protection personnel are true?
   A. The radiation protection advisor is normally responsible for day-to-day management of radiation protection
   B. The radiation protection supervisor has overall responsibility for radiation protection
   C. All medical physics experts are radiation protection advisors
   D. The radiation protection advisor is normally responsible for carrying out a risk assessment on new X-ray equipment
   E. The radiation protection supervisor is normally responsible for carrying out checks on personal protective equipment

---

Many people are involved in the supervision of radiation protection. The Ionising Radiations Regulations (1999) require a radiation protection advisor to be consulted on compliance with regulations. The radiation protection advisor is normally responsible for making risk assessment on new equipment or new radiopharmaceutical use, and advising the employer on compliance with radiation regulations. Medical physics experts are required under the Ionising Radiation (Medical Exposure) Regulations (2000) who are involved with optimization and quality control. Radiation protection advisors often also act as medical physics experts, however this is not always the case. The radiation protection supervisor is normally responsible for checking personal radiation equipment, supervising staff monitoring, investigating excessive doses and preparing local rules. The radiation protection supervisor is normally responsible for day-to-day management of radiation protection however it is the employer that has overall responsibility for radiation protection.

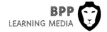

9.   A.   **False** – the radiation protection supervisor is normally responsible for day-to-day management of radiation protection

B.   **False** – the employer has overall responsibility for radiation protection

C.   **False** – not all medical physics experts are radiation protection advisors

D.   **True** – the radiation protection advisor is normally responsible for carrying out a risk assessment on new X-ray equipment

E.   **True** – the radiation protection supervisor is normally responsible for carrying out checks on personal protective equipment

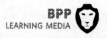

10. Regarding notifiable incidents under IRR 99
    A. If a woman receives 10 times the intended dose for a mammogram due to equipment failure the Care Quality Commission should be notified
    B. A radiation source being stolen is a notifiable incident
    C. If there is a minor radiation source spillage this is a notifiable incident
    D. If the abdomen of a woman of reproductive capacity receives more than 13 mSv in 3 months this is a notifiable incident
    E. An overexposure of greater than 1.5 times the intended dose of a barium swallow due to a fault in the automatic exposure control system is a notifiable incident

The Ionising Radiation Regulations (1999) describe certain events when the Health and Safety Executive should be notified. These include a radiation source being lost, stolen or spilt causing significant contamination (a small spill does not need to be reported to the Health and Safety Executive). If any dose limit is exceeded including that of a member of public then it must be reported. Finally if a patient receives a dose much greater than intended it must be reported. This varies depending on what imaging or radiological procedure is being done. For example the guidance figure for overexposure of mammograms is 10 times the intended dose. Overexposure by greater than 1.5 times the intended dose of interventional radiology, radiographic and fluoroscopic procedures involving contrast agents, CT examinations or high-dose nuclear medicine procedure are all notifiable.

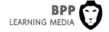

10. A. **False** – if a woman receives 10 times the intended dose for a mammogram due to equipment failure the Health and Safety Executive should be notified

B. **True** – a radiation source being stolen is a notifiable incident

C. **False** – if there is a minor radiation source spillage this is not necessarily a notifiable incident

D. **True** – if the abdomen of a woman of reproductive capacity receives more than 13 mSv in 3 months this is a notifiable incident

E. **True** – an overexposure of greater than 1.5 times the intended dose of a barium swallow due to a fault in the automatic exposure control system is a notifiable incident

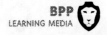

11. Regarding basic radiation protection principles
    A. When deciding on whether an examination is justified, the ALARP principle should be taken into account
    B. The recommendations of the International Commission on Radiological Protection introduced three basic principles of radiation protection: justification, optimisation and diagnostic reference levels
    C. Justification can be made where the medical benefit does not exceed the risk
    D. Radiation protection is considered appropriate if exposure is kept within the required limits
    E. Dose limits do not apply to patients

The three basic principles of radiation protection of justification, optimisation and dose limitation were set out by the International Commission on Radiological Protection (1991).

Justification of the use of ionising radiation is decided on whether the benefits outweigh the risks. These benefits do not necessarily have to be for the medical health of the individual; they could be for economic reasons such as radiation doses to nuclear power workers, or in medical trials when society in general may benefit.

Optimization is the process whereby the dose is kept as low as reasonably practical (ALARP) and this can involve both the technology used and the operator technique.

Dose limits are used to limit the number of stochastic and deterministic effects of radiation on staff and members of the public. Compliance with limits does not get rid of the need for doses to be kept as low as practicably possible in accordance with optimisation. Patient dose is not subject to dose limits, this is only determined by justification and optimisation.

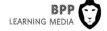

11. A. **False** – the ALARP principle should be taken into account in optimisation
    B. **False** – diagnostic reference levels are part of the requirements of Ionising Radiation (Medical Exposure) Regulation 2000
    C. **True** – justification can be made where the medical benefit does not exceed the risk
    D. **False** – doses still need to be keep as low as reasonably possible
    E. **True** – dose limits do not apply to patients

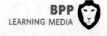

12. Regarding the ionising radiation regulations
   A. The Ionising Radiation Regulations (1999) set out the roles of referrer, practitioner and operator
   B. The Ionising Radiation (Medical Exposure) Regulations (2000) require dose limits to be defined for different procedures
   C. Classification of persons is required under the Ionising Radiation Regulations (1999)
   D. The Radioactive Substances Act (1993) requires users of radioactive sources to be registered and licensed
   E. The Medicines (Administration of Radioactive Substances) Regulations (1978) introduced a system of licensed disposal sources

The Ionising Radiations Regulations (1999) has a number of requirements including consultation with a radiation protection advisor; notification of the Health and Safety Executive of use of ionising radiation; introducing dose limits; designation of controlled and supervised areas; classification of staff; and reasons to notify the Health and Safety Executive.

The Ionising Radiation (Medical Exposure) Regulations (2000) sets out the referrer, practitioner and operator roles, requires diagnostic reference levels for examinations and requires advice of a medical physics expert.

The Radioactive Substances Act (1993) sets out a system of licensing and registration for users of radioactive sources and licensed disposal routes.

The Medicines (Administration of Radioactive Substances) Regulations (1978) require doctors who inject radioactive substances to have a certificate for each specific procedure which is issued by the Administration of Radioactive Substances Advisory Committee.

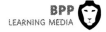

12. A. **False** – the Ionising Radiation (Medical Exposure) Regulations (2000) set out the roles of referrer, practitioner and operator
    B. **False** – the Ionising Radiations Regulations (1999) require dose limits to be defined for different procedures
    C. **True** – classification of persons is required under the Ionising Radiation Regulations (1999)
    D. **True** – the Radioactive Substances Act (1993) requires users of radioactive sources to be registered and licensed
    E. **False** – the Radioactive Substances Act (1993) introduces a system of licensed disposal sources

13. Which of the following statements regarding designated work areas are correct?
    A. Designation of supervised areas is a requirement of the Ionising Radiation (Medical Exposure) Regulations 2001
    B. A supervised area is one in which the person working in the area is likely to receive a radiation dose greater than $\frac{3}{10}$ of any dose limit
    C. A controlled area is an area in which the external dose rate could exceed over 7.5 μSvhr^{-1} averaged over the working day
    D. A waiting area for people who have been injected with a radiopharmaceutical is likely to be a controlled area
    E. Controlled areas must be clearly marked with warning signs

The Ionising Radiations Regulations (1999) require designation of radiation areas and procedures. Radiation areas are split into supervised and controlled areas. A supervised area is an area where it is likely a person could exceed the annual dose limit for a member of the public, or where it is necessary to keep the area under review in case it may need to be designated a controlled area.

A controlled area is an area where a person is likely to receive greater than $\frac{3}{10}$ of any dose limit, there is a requirement to follow special procedures to restrict exposure, or where the external dose rate could exceed over 7.5 μSvhr^{-1} averaged over the working day. Controlled areas must be marked with signs describing the nature of the radiation. For mobile X-rays the controlled area is generally considered to be the area 2 m from the X-ray tube, with verbal warning given by the radiographer. An area where people are injected with a radiopharmaceutical is likely to be a controlled area; one where they are waiting post-injection is likely to be a supervised area.

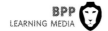

13. A. **False** – designation of supervised areas is a requirement of the Ionising Radiations Regulations (1999)

B. **False** – a controlled area is one in which the person working in the area is likely to receive a radiation dose greater than $\frac{3}{10}$ of any dose limit

C. **True** – a controlled area is also an area in which the external dose rate could exceed over 7.5 μSvhr^{-1} averaged over the working day

D. **False** – a waiting area for people who have been injected with a radiopharmaceutical is likely to be a supervised area

E. **True** – controlled areas must be clearly marked with warning signs

14. Which of the following statements regarding the policing bodies relevant to radiology in the UK are correct?
   A. The enforcing agency for regulations under the Health and Safety at Work Act is the Health and Safety Commission
   B. The enforcing agency for the regulations under the Ionising Radiations Regulations is the Health and Safety Executive
   C. The enforcing agency for the Ionising Radiation (Medical Exposure) Regulations is the Healthcare Commission
   D. The enforcing agency for the Radioactive Substances Act is the Administration of Radioactive Substances Advisory Committee
   E. The enforcing agency for the Medicines (Administration of Radioactive Substances) Regulations is the Department of Health

There are several advisory and enforcing bodies concerned with ionising radiation.

The Health and Safety at Work Act (1974) set up an advisory body, the Health and Safety Commission, and an enforcing body, the Health and Safety Executive. This means the Ionising Radiations Regulations (1999) are enforced by the Health and Safety Executive.

Confusingly, despite the Ionising Radiation (Medical Exposure) Regulations (2000) coming under the Health and Safety Act, it is enforced by the Healthcare Commission.

The Environmental Agency enforces the Radioactive Substances Act (1993) as this concerns licenses to hold and dispose of radioactive substances.

The Medicines (Administration of Radioactive Substances) Regulations (1978) are enforced by the Administration of Radioactive Substances Advisory Committee, which itself is a branch of the Department of Health. They give certificates granting a license

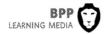

for doctors to perform certain procedures which involve giving patients radioactive products.

---

14. A. **False** – the enforcing agency for regulations under the Health and Safety at Work Act is the Health and Safety Executive
     B. **True** – the enforcing agency for the regulations under the Ionising Radiations Regulations is the Health and Safety Executive
     C. **True** – the enforcing agency for the Ionising Radiation (Medical Exposure) Regulations is the Healthcare Commission
     D. **False** – the enforcing agency for the Radioactive Substances Act is the Environmental Agency
     E. **True** – the enforcing agency for the Medicines (Administration of Radioactive Substances) Regulations is the Department of Health

15. With regard to the classification of people under IRR (1999)
 A. Classification is required for any person whose dose is likely to exceed the dose limit
 B. Once classified, the employee needs to go for monthly health checks
 C. Most radiographers are designated as classified workers
 D. The Ionising Radiation Regulations 1999 require all staff exposed to radiation to undergo dose monitoring
 E. A 17-year-old employee cannot become a classified worker

Classification of persons is required under the Ionising Radiation Regulations (1999) for any person whose dose is likely to exceed $\frac{3}{10}$ of any dose limit to identify those at risk from the effects of radiation. Classified workers need to go for annual health checks, the records of which are held for 50 years. The Ionising Radiation Regulations require only classified staff to undergo monitoring, however the employer is required to show that the dose to other staff working within controlled areas is adequately controlled, hence most staff have some form of monitoring. Only individuals who are 18 years old or over, and certified medically fit to practice, can be classified workers. Radiographers are rarely designated as classified workers. The most likely staff to be classified are interventional radiologists and cardiologists.

---

15. A. **False** – classification is required for any person whose dose is likely to exceed $\frac{3}{10}$ of the dose limit
 B. **False** – classified employees need to go for annual health checks
 C. **False** – radiographers are rarely designated as classified workers
 D. **False** – the Ionising Radiation Regulations 1999 require classified staff to undergo dose monitoring
 E. **True** – a 17-year-old employee cannot become a classified worker

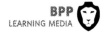

16. Which of the following statements regarding the various roles detailed by IRMER are correct?
    A. The referrer is responsible for justifying the examination
    B. The person in the practitioner role is responsible for performing the examination
    C. The same person can be practitioner and operator
    D. The referrer must have a medical or dental degree
    E. The operator does not need to be a health professional

The three main roles for people involved in a medical radiation exposure are set out by the Ionising Radiation (Medical Exposure) Regulations (2000). The referrer is the person who requests the X-ray. The employer is responsible for defining who can request radiographic examinations. Healthcare professionals other than doctors may also have been trained to act as referrers depending on local rules determined by the employer, for example physiotherapists or nurse practictioners may be able to order certain radiographs.

The practitioner is responsible for weighing up the associated risks and benefits of an examination and ultimately justifying it. Again, the employer must define who is able to act in this capacity but it is normally someone that has acquired knowledge of ionising radiation, protection and techniques. This is normally a radiologist or radiographer, but other healthcare professionals such as cardiologists or dentists may act in this role.

The operator role is used to designate a person involved in the practical exposure of the patient, for example the radiographer performing an examination. There is no requirement for the operator to be a healthcare professional, as technicians or engineers performing maintenance are also classified as operators. An individual may perform duties of both practitioner and operator – for example a radiographer may be able to act as a practitioner depending on local rules.

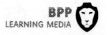

16. A. **False** – the practitioner is responsible for justifying the examination
    B. **False** – the person in the operator role is the person responsible for performing the examination
    C. **True** – the same person can be practitioner and operator
    D. **False** – the referrer does not need to have a medical or dental degree
    E. **True** – the operator does not need to be a healthcare professional

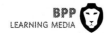

17. Which of the typical effective doses and investigations given below are correctly paired?
  A. A CT abdomen has a typical effective dose of 10 mSv
  B. A barium enema has a typical effective dose of 3 mSv
  C. A CT head has a typical effective dose of 5 mSv
  D. A PA chest film has a typical effective dose of 0.15 mSv
  E. A lung perfusion study has a typical effective dose of 1 mSv

---

A CT abdomen or pelvis has a typical effective dose of 10 mSv. CT of the chest has a typical effective dose of 8 mSv. A CT head has a typical effective dose of 2 mSv. Using two plain films to examine the head has a typical effective dose of 0.04 mSv. A lung perfusion study has a typical effective dose of 1 mSv. A barium enema has a typical effective dose of 7 mSv, while a barium meal has a typical effective dose of 3 mSv and a barium swallow has a typical effective dose of 1.5 mSv. The absorbed dose of a PA chest film is 0.15 mSv, the typical effective dose is 0.015 mSv.

---

17. A. **True** – a CT abdomen has a typical effective dose of 10 mSv
  B. **False** – a barium enema has a typical effective dose of 7 mSv
  C. **False** – a CT head has a typical effective dose of 2 mSv
  D. **False** – a PA chest film has a typical effective dose of 0.015 mSv
  E. **True** – a lung perfusion study has a typical effective dose of 1 mSv

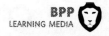

18. Regarding staff protection
    A. 12 cm of solid brick will provide equivalent protection of 1 mm of lead
    B. An under-couch tube is preferable to an over-couch tube
    C. Lead aprons generally provide equivalent protection of 2.5–5 mm lead
    D. Lead aprons will provide adequate protection from the primary beam
    E. Minimising exposure time and maximising distance from the X-tube will reduce dose

---

The design of the X-ray exposure room is important to minimise the spread of ionising radiation. In newer construction buildings lead sheets 1–2 mm thick are incorporated into the walls. 120 mm of normal solid brick will provide equivalent protection of 1 mm of lead. Personal protection is necessary to provide protection for staff working in the unprotected parts of the controlled area rooms. Lead aprons generally incorporate between 0.25–0.5 mm lead, and are designed to provide protection from scattered radiation but do not provide adequate protection from the primary beam. An under-couch tube is generally always preferable to an over-couch tube. The entrance scatter will be much higher than the exit scatter so it is preferable this occurs to the lower extremities rather than the more radiosensitive upper extremities.

---

18. A. **False** – 12 mm of solid brick will provide equivalent protection of 1 mm of lead
    B. **True** – an undercouch tube is preferable to an overcouch tube
    C. **False** – lead aprons generally provide equivalent protection of 0.25–0.5 mm lead
    D. **False** – lead aprons will not provide adequate protection from the primary beam
    E. **True** – minimising exposure time and maximising distance from the X-tube will reduce dose

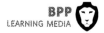

Chapter 14

MRI physics

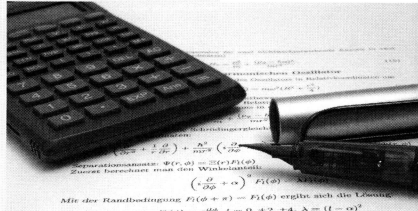

MRI physics

Please answer all questions true or false. There is no negative marking.

---

1. Regarding MRI
   A. T1 recovery involves the transfer of energy to surrounding environment
   B. The T1 time of fat is longer than that of water
   C. T2 decay is predominantly due to external magnetic field inhomogeneities
   D. Long TE maximises the T2 contrast between fat and water
   E. Proton density weighting attempts to diminish T1 and T2 effects

---

After a radio frequency pulse at the Larmor frequency has been applied and removed, relaxation processes occur resulting in a decrease in the amplitude of the net magnetic vector in the transverse plane. Thus the voltage measured by the receiver coil decreases (known as free induction decay).

Spin-lattice energy transfer: this reflects nuclei shifting their magnetic moments from high- to low- energy states, with the energy exchanged to their surrounding environment. T1 recovery is a reflection of the efficiency of this exponential process (time taken for 63% of **longitudinal** magnetisation to recover). Fat is able to absorb energy quickly and T1 is short; water is inefficient at receiving energy from nuclei so T1 is longer.

Loss of precessional coherence: NMV decays in **transverse** plane by:

- **Spin-spin energy transfer**: interactions of the intrinsic magnetic fields of adjacent nuclei. This is described by T2 decay (time for 63% of transverse magnetisation to be lost due to dephasing). Fat is much better at this energy exchange

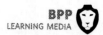

than water (molecular motion matches Larmor frequency better) so T2 time is short.

- **Inhomogeneities of external magnetic field**: these are inevitable in current magnets. As magnetic field strength is part of the Larmor equation, nuclei within inhomogeneities will precess at slightly different frequencies and diphase. This exponential process is known as T2* decay and precedes T2 decay 'proper'.

The TR controls how much of the longitudinal NMV in fat or water has recovered before the next RF pulse (thus how much differential T1 contrast is seen diminishes over time). The TE controls how much transverse magnetisation has been allowed to decay in fat and water when the signal is read (T2 contrast – exaggerated over time). Long TEs allow dephasing of the transverse components in fat and water, so demonstrating a contrast difference.

Proton density weighting seeks to diminish the effects of differences in T1 recovery and T2 decay within tissues, to produce an image whose contrast is predominantly due to differences in proton density (ie long TR and short TE).

---

1. A. **True** – T1 recovery is concerned with spin lattice energy transfer
    B. **False** – water is inefficient at receiving energy from nuclei so T1 is longer
    C. **False** – T2 decay is due to spin-spin energy transfer, field inhomogeneities are responsible for T2* decay
    D. **True** – long TE maximises contrast between fat and water
    E. **True** – this is the purpose of PD weighting

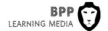

> 2. Regarding MRI sequences
>   A. Gradient echo may produce T2 weighted images
>   B. In T2 weighted fast/turbo spin echo, water and fat are hyperintense
>   C. Spins may be rephased by using a '180 degree' RF pulse
>   D. Gradient echo uses an RF pulse to rephase spins in a pulse sequence
>   E. Signal-to-noise ratio in gradient echo is less than in spin echo sequence

---

Pulse sequences describe the way in which the MRI system applies RF pulses and gradients (and intervening timings) and thus controls weighting of the image.

Inhomogeneities in the magnetic field cause rapid dephasing and necessitate pulse sequences to rephase spins and remove inhomogeneity effects (and thus truly reflect tissue decay characteristics), as well as enable manipulation of the TE and TR. Conventional spin echo sequences use a 90degree excitation pulse followed by a 180 degree rephasing pulse (or several pulses) which regenerate signal in the receiver coil from that generated by the initial RF pulse (hence the term 'spin echo').

Fast/turbo spin echo represents an attempt to speed up conventional spin echo by using a single RF excitation pulse followed by a train of 180 degree rephasing pulses (each followed by phase encoding and data acquisition). The succession of 180 degree pulses reduces the spin-spin interactions in fat, thereby increasing its T2 decay time – so fat may appear bright on T2 weighted images in FSE.

Gradient echo sequences by definition use the gradient coils to rephase spins. This is less efficient at eliminating the effects of $T2^*$ decay; hence when attempting to maximise T2 decay contrast within tissues, gradient echo sequences are described as producing $T2^*$ weighted images. In gradient echo, a flip angle other than 90 degrees is used, so only part of the longitudinal magnetisation is converted to transverse magnetisation. As a result SNR is less than in spin echo sequences.

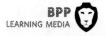

2.   A.   **False** – owing to field inhomogeneity susceptibility only T2* weighting is achieved
     B.   **True** – water and fat are hyperintense in T2 weighted FSE
     C.   **True** – this is the purpose of the 180 degree RF pulse
     D.   **False** – GE sequences use gradient coils to rephase spins
     E.   **True** – in GE sequences only part of the longitudinal magnetisation is converted to transverse magnetisation as a result SNR is less than in spin echo sequences

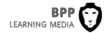

3. Regarding MRI sequences
   A. In conventional spin echo the TR is the time from one 90 degree RF pulse to the next 90 degree RF excitation pulse
   B. In spin echo magnetic field inhomogeneities are eliminated
   C. Inversion recovery using short time to inversion (TI) allows suppression of the signal from CSF
   D. In gradient echo rephasing is usually performed by the phase encoding gradient
   E. In gradient echo a small 'flip angle' is required for T1 weighting

In conventional spin echo, after application of a 90 degree RF excitation pulse spins lose precessional coherence because of magnetic field inhomogeneities. A 180 degree RF pulse then flips the dephased nuclei through 180 degrees and rephases them – effectively eliminating the effect of magnetic inhomogeneities. The TR is the length of time from one 90 degree RF pulse to the next. The TE is the length of time from the 90 degree RF pulse to the mid-point or peak of the signal generated after the 180 degree RF pulse.

Inversion recovery (IR) is a spin echo sequence beginning with a 180 degree inverting pulse (TR is the time between *these* pulses in IR), followed by a 90 degree pulse at time interval TI and a further 180 degree rephasing pulse. (TE is defined as same as in conventional spin echo). TI controls weighting. Tissue signal may be suppressed if the 90 degree RF pulse coincides with the time at which a tissue's NMV is passing exactly through the transverse plane after the initial 180 degree inverting pulse; the 90 degree pulse then 'pushes' this to 180 degrees, and therefore the tissue produces no transverse component. The time for this is short for fat (100–180 ms) and results in fat suppression (short TI inversion recovery- STIR), and long for fluid (1700–2200 ms).

Gradient echo uses a gradient (typically the frequency encoding gradient) to reduce magnetic homogeneity effects. Weighting is controlled by the TR and TE (as previously), as well as the degree to

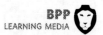

which the longitudinal magnetisation is converted to the transverse plane (the flip angle). For T1 weighting the majority of the NMV must be shifted towards the transverse plane so a large flip angle must be used (with a short TR and short TE).

---

3. A. **True** – by definition
    B. **True** – this is performed by the 180 degree RF pulse rephasing
    C. **False** – STIR sequences suppress the signal from fat
    D. **False** – rephasing in GE is usually performed by the frequency encoding gradient
    E. **False** – in GE sequences T1 weighting uses a large flip angle to shift the NMV towards the transverse plane

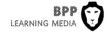

4. Regarding MRI gradients and image production
    A. Gradient coils change the field strength across a distance in the patient in an exponential fashion
    B. Gradient coils enable slice selection
    C. Phase encoding gradients are used to locate signal along the short axis
    D. K space does not correspond directly with MR images
    E. Decreasing the frequency matrix increases the minimum TE

Gradients are coils of wire that alter the magnetic field of the magnet in a linear fashion when a current is passed through them. They are usually situated deep to the RF coils. By changing the magnetic field strength in a predictable fashion, they change the precessional frequency (encoding the long axis) and phase (encoding the short axis) of magnetic moments of nuclei, and enable encoding of the MR signal in three dimensions.

The slice select gradient is switched on during the delivery of the RF excitation pulse (3.2 ms in the positive direction). Phase encoding gradient is switched on after the RF excitation pulse has been switched off (4 ms). The frequency encoding gradient is switched on during the echo (8 ms).

K space is a spatial frequency domain where data from the signal are stored; it does not correspond to final MR images.

The number of data points in each line of K space corresponds to the frequency matrix (eg 256 or 512); increasing the frequency matrix or reducing the receive bandwidth increase the minimum TE (as dictated by the Nyquist theorem).

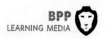

4.   A.   **False** – gradient coils change the field strength in a linear fashion

       B.   **True** – gradient coils are the primary means of slice selection

       C.   **True** – phase encoding is used to locate signal in the short axis

       D.   **True** – K space is merely a storage concept

       E.   **False** – increasing the frequency matrix increases the minimum TE

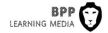

5.   Regarding MRI image quality
     A.   Agents which shorten T1 worsen image contrast
     B.   Decreasing TE will improve signal-to-noise ratio
     C.   Increasing matrix size decreases spatial resolution
     D.   Increasing field strength improves signal-to-noise ratio
     E.   Reducing TR decreases scan time

Signal-to-noise ratio (SNR) is the ratio of useful MR signal to background noise. SNR is increased by increasing field strength, using phased coil arrays, long TR, short TE, large flip angles, increasing number of signal averages, reducing received bandwidth and imaging proton dense structures. All these measures will increase the amplitude and/or duration of the transverse magnetisation component; thus maximising the voltage induced in the receiver coil.

Contrast agents such as gadolinium shorten T1 in lesions. These appear bright on T1 weighting and therefore SNR is improved.

Spatial resolution is controlled by the size of the voxel. Decreasing voxel size increases spatial resolution (at the expense of SNR), thus increasing matrix size, decreasing slice thickness or decreasing field of view will increase spatial resolution.

Scan time is the product of TR, number of phase encodings and number of signal averages (and in fast scanning, the number of slice encodings). Reducing TR thus decreases scan time, but will also reduce SNR and the number of slices available.

5.   A.   **False** – contrast agents such as gadolinium shorten T1 and increase SNR
     B.   **True** – short TE improves SNR
     C.   **False** – this will decrease voxel size and increase spatial resolution
     D.   **True** – will increase useful signal received over noise
     E.   **True** – scan time is dependent on TR

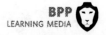

6.   Regarding MRI
      A.   Hydrogen nuclei resonate at the same frequency in different body tissues
      B.   Magnetic susceptibility artefact may occur in association with prostheses
      C.   Motion artefact affects the frequency encoding axis
      D.   Flowing blood usually appears dark with spin echo sequences
      E.   Gadolinium is a super–paramagnetic agent

In water hydrogen is linked to oxygen, and in fat it is linked to carbon. These chemically different environments cause hydrogen nuclei to have different precessional frequencies in these two molecules (hydrogen in fat resonates at a lower frequency than water). This may result in the artefact of chemical shift—a signal void between areas of fat and water. This is made worse by increasing magnetic field strength or narrowing the receive bandwidth. It occurs in the frequency-encoding axis, whereas most other artefacts tend to affect the phase encoding axis.

Magnetic susceptibility occurs because tissues magnetise to differing degrees and so have differing individual precessional frequency and phase. It is most pronounced at the boundaries of structures with the greatest disparity - for example with metal prostheses. It may be partially remedied by using sequences that use RF rephasing (SE), or by removing metal items.

Motion artefact (also known as phase mismapping) results from tissue movement between the application of the phase encoding gradient and the frequency encoding gradient, or motion between each application of the phase gradient. The tissue is thereby assigned the wrong phase value and is mismapped (appearing blurred or ghosted).

Spin echo sequences will usually show a signal void with blood flowing through vessels (gradient echo, in contrast, will show a bright signal).

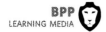

Gadolinium is a paramagnetic agent that has seven unpaired electrons allowing rapid exchange of bulk water to minimise the space between itself and water, reducing T1 relaxation time. It is used as a T1 contrast enhancement agent (often in neuroradiology). Iron oxides are super paramagnetic substances that shorten T2 times.

---

6.   A.   **False** – this is demonstrated in chemical shift artefact

        B.   **True** – the effect may be pronounced around prostheses

        C.   **False** – motion artefact affects the phase encoding axis

        D.   **True** – spin echo sequences show a signal void with flowing blood

        E.   **False** – gadolinium is a paramagnetic agent

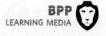

7. Regarding MRI design
    A. Scanners using permanent magnets do not allow open design
    B. Superconducting electromagnets used in scanners must be kept at absolute zero
    C. Shim coils are used to improve field homogeneity
    D. Phased array radiofrequency coils degrade SNR
    E. One Tesla magnetic field is 200 times the Earth's magnetic field strength

Permanent magnets are ferromagnetic substances that have a magnetic susceptibility >1 (eg iron or nickel). They retain magnetisation and allow open design and require no power supply; however they are heavy, and can only provide low fixed field strengths. Modern MRI scanners utilise superconducting electromagnets whose resistance decreases with decreasing temperature, thus allowing the energy required to maintain the field to be minimised. The coils are 'ramped' up by the application of current and creation of an electric field; they are then supercooled with cryogens (eg liquid helium) to eliminate resistance. This cooling approaches a few degrees of absolute zero (-273 degrees Celsius or 0 degrees Kelvin) but does not reach this.

Magnet field inhomogeneities are unavoidable in scanners, as electromagnet coils cannot be evenly spaced. Current carrying (shim) coils are placed in the area of inhomogeneity to even this out. Inhomogeneities are measured in parts-per-million and homogeneity of below approximately 10 ppm is required for conventional imaging.

Radiofrequency coils produce a magnetic field at 90 degrees to the bore magnetic field produced by the magnet. Phased array coils are multiple coils and receivers where individual signals are combined to create one image with improved SNR and coverage.

One Tesla is equivalent to 10,000 Gauss. The Earth's magnetic field is 0.5 Gauss; therefore one Tesla is 20,000 times this.

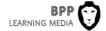

7.   A.   **False** – permanent magnets allow open design
      B.   **False** – superconducting electromagnets are kept a few degrees above absolute zero
      C.   **True** – shim coils smooth the external magnetic field inhomogeneities
      D.   **False** – phased array coils are used to improve SNR
      E.   **False** – one Tesla is equivalent to 20,000 times the Earth's magnetic field

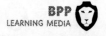

8.   The Larmor frequency is
        A.   Proportionate to the applied magnetic field
        B.   The same for each hydrogen atom within all
             tissues
        C.   The frequency of the applied radiofrequency pulse
        D.   Inversely proportional to the gyromagnetic ratio
        E.   Constant with varying external magnetic field
             strengths

The Larmor equation provides the frequency (or precessional speed)
for a specific nucleus in a given magnetic field as follows:

$$\textsf{l}_0 = B_0 \times ©$$

where $\textsf{l}_0$ denotes precessional frequency, B_0 is the strength of
the external magnetic field, and © or gyromagnetic ratio is the
precessional frequency of a given nucleus at 1 Tesla (MHz/T).

The Larmor frequency for hydrogen nuclei varies, depending on
what atoms they are chemically linked to (eg in water and fat) and
this phenomenon is responsible for chemical shift artefact.

8.   A.   **True** – as defined by the Larmor equation
        B.   **False** – the precessional frequency for hydrogen nuclei
                     varies depending on the atoms with which they
                     are linked
        C.   **True** – the frequency of the applied radiofrequency
                     pulse is derived from the Larmor equation and
                     causes coherence of the magnetic moments of
                     hydrogen and gives a measurable voltage on
                     detection
        D.   **False** – Larmor frequency is directly proportional to
                     gyromagnetic ration
        E.   **False** – Larmor frequency is directly proportional to
                     field strength

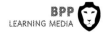

> 9. Regarding MRI
>   A. Only signals from hydrogen may be used
>   B. Can be used to demonstrate blood flow
>   C. Demonstrates that T1 is longer than T2 in biological tissues
>   D. Spin lattice energy transfer is inefficient in water
>   E. Cortical bone is dark on proton density weighting

Protons and neutrons within a nucleus spin about their own axes in a random fashion (clockwise or anticlockwise); when there are an equal number of spinning nucleons they will tend to cancel one another out. A nucleus with an odd mass number will have net spin, and (given that protons have charge) net charge. A moving unbalanced charge induces a magnetic field, and this forms the basis of MR imaging.

Flowing blood within a vessel may be described as laminar (or first order with blood flowing at variable but consistent velocities across the lumen), turbulent (randomly fluctuating), or vortex (as through a stricture).

First order flow may be compensated for. Various techniques may be employed to image flowing blood. For example, 'bright blood' imaging uses gradient moment nulling (with coherent gradient echo sequences) to make flowing blood bright. Time of flight angiography (TOF-MRA) produces vascular contrast by varying longitudinal magnetisation of stationary spins in gradient echo spins sequences, in such a way that the TR is kept below the T1 time of the stationary tissues. (T1 recovery is prevented.) Fully magnetised flowing 'fresh' spins produce high signal and hence high contrast is attained. Phase-contrast MRA (PC-MRA) relies on velocity changes and thus phase shifts in moving spins to provide image contrast in flowing vessels.

T1 recovery time of a particular tissue is caused by 'spin lattice' energy transfer from nuclei to their surrounding environment and defined as time taken for 63% 'recovery' of the longitudinal NMV. In contrast, T2 decay reflects exchange of energy from one nucleus to another as a result of spin-spin energy transfer and magnetic field

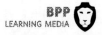

inhomogeneities. Defined as time taken for 63% of the transverse magnetisation to 'decay', this inherently takes less time than T1 recovery and is reflected in the fact that TR is longer than TE.

PD weighted images demonstrate differences in proton densities within the FOV by diminishing both T1 and T2 effects; this is achieved by using a long TR and short TE. PD weighting is useful in showing anatomy and some pathology. Tissues with low proton density are dark as a result of a small transverse magnetisation. Examples of this are seen when imaging cortical bone and air.

---

9. A. **False** – nuclei with an odd number of nucleons (mass number) are MR active and can be used to form images
   B. **True** – blood flow may give rise to characteristic (and therefore recognisable) artefact or can be targeted with specific sequences
   C. **True** – T1 recovery is always longer than T2 decay in biological tissues
   D. **True** – spin lattice energy transfer is synonymous with T1 recovery, water is inefficient at receiving energy from other nuclei
   E. **True** – low proton density structures are dark on PD weighted images

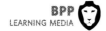

10. Regarding MRI safety
   A. Static magnetic field bioeffects may include heating of patients and hypotension
   B. Gradient time-varying fields can cause cardiac arrhythmias
   C. Presence of cochlear implant is a relative contraindication to MRI
   D. Most orthopaedic implants show no deflection within the main magnet
   E. MRI scanning is contraindicated in the first trimester of pregnancy

The potential for harm in MRI may be considered to be due to the effects of the static magnetic field generated by the magnetic coils and the effects of oscillating gradients. The static field is effectively permanent (unless the coils are quenched) and may extend beyond the examination room; bioeffects are reversible and may include heating of patients, headaches, fatigue, hypotension and hydrodynamic effects (eg ECG changes).

The bioeffects of time-varying gradients occur only during sequences; changes in magnetic field induce currents which can affect tissues that act as conductors (eg nerves and muscles). Visual disturbance, cutaneous sensory disturbances, muscle fasciculation and cardiac arrhythmias may result with gradients.

Implants and prostheses must be considered when determining patient suitability for MR scanning. Ferromagnetic items of clinical equipment must not be brought into the scan room. Cardiac pacemakers, implanted insulin pumps, nerve stimulators and cochlear implants are absolute contraindications for MR scanning. Intra-ocular ferrous foreign bodies must be excluded. Orthopaedic implants usually are not deflected within the main magnet; however in larger prostheses induced currents can generate heat. (This is relatively low, however).

There are no proven bioeffects of MR scanning on foetuses; theoretical risks have been described. There are no official guidelines, though due to these theoretical considerations it is suggested that MRI be

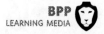

delayed past the first trimester if possible. This is not absolute and would depend on the clinical situation.

---

10. A. **True** – the static field carries the risk of reversible abnormalities including patient heating and hypotension

B. **True** – oscillating gradients can induce currents in nerves and blood vessels which have the potential to cause cardiac arrhythmias

C. **False** – presence of cochlear implants is an absolute contraindication to MRI, being attracted to the magnetic field and being operationally dependent on magnetic or electronic activation

D. **True** – most orthopaedic implants are not deflected within the field

E. **False** – there are no official guidelines; it is recommended that scanning should be delayed if possible until after the first trimester, if clinically possible

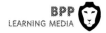

11. Regarding MRI gradient echo sequences
   A. In gradient echo sequences the flip angle is independent of the magnitude of the radiofrequency excitation pulse
   B. In gradient echo the TE controls T2 weighting
   C. In gradient echo rephasing is performed by the frequency encoding gradient
   D. Gradient echo images are less sensitive to external magnetic field inhomogeneities
   E. The pulse control unit synchronises the application of gradients and radiofrequency pulses in a pulse sequence

Gradient echo uses a gradient (typically the frequency encoding gradient) to reduce magnetic homogeneity effects. Weighting is controlled by the TR and TE (as previously) as well as the degree to which the longitudinal magnetisation is converted to the transverse plane (the flip angle). The flip angle is dependent on the magnitude and duration of the RF excitation pulse. For T1 weighting the majority of the NMV must be shifted towards the transverse plane, so a large flip angle must be used (with a short TR and short TE). Increased susceptibility to external magnetic field inhomogeneity means that $T2^*$ weighting may achieved and is dependent on TE.

11. A. **False** – the flip angle is dependent on the magnitude and duration of the RF excitation pulse
   B. **False** – in gradient echo, TE controls $T2^*$ weighting
   C. **True** – gradient echo employs the frequency encoding gradient for rephasing
   D. **False** – gradient echo images are more sensitive to external field inhomogeneity due to $T2^*$ dephasing effects
   E. **True** – the pulse control unit synchronises the gradients and RF pulses in a sequence

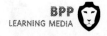

> 12. Regarding MRI sequences
>   A. In conventional spin echo a short TR is used to produce T1 weighting
>   B. Short time to inversion sequences (STIR) use 180 degree pulses to rephase spins
>   C. T2 weighting is achieved by using a long TE
>   D. Oedema is typically bright on T2 weighted images
>   E. Fluid attenuated inversion recovery (FLAIR) sequences typically use time to inversion (TI) times in excess of one second

In conventional spin echo, after application of a 90 degree RF excitation pulse spins lose precessional coherence because of magnetic field inhomogeneities. A 180 degree RF pulse then flips the dephased nuclei through 180 degrees and rephases them – effectively eliminating the effect of magnetic inhomogeneities. The TR is the length of time from one 90 degree RF pulse to the next. The TE is the length of time from the 90 degree RF pulse to the mid-point or peak of the signal generated after the 180 degree RF pulse.

T1 weighting requires short TR and TE.

Inversion recovery (IR) is a spin echo sequence beginning with a 180 degree inverting pulse (TR is the time between *these* pulses in IR), followed by a 90 degree pulse at time interval TI and a further 180 degree rephasing pulse. (TE is defined as same as in conventional spin echo). TI controls weighting. Tissue signal may be suppressed if the 90 degree RF pulse coincides with the time at which a tissue's NMV is passing exactly through the transverse plane after the initial 180 degree inverting pulse; the 90 degree pulse then 'pushes' this to 180 degrees, and therefore the tissue produces no transverse component. The time for this is short for fat (100-180 ms) and results in fat suppression (short TI inversion recovery- STIR), and long for fluid (1700-2200 ms).

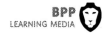

12. A. **True** – in conventional spin echo T1 weighting is achieved using a short TR
    B. **True** – inversion recovery sequences use 180 degree pulses to rephase spins
    C. **True** – T2 weighted images are achieved using long TE
    D. **True** – water is bright on T2 weighted images
    E. **True** – FLAIR uses long TIs of 1700–2200 ms to null signal from CSF (which has a long T1 recovery time)

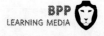

13. Regarding MRI
    A. The time constant T2 is the time it takes for 50% of the transverse magnetisation to be lost
    B. T1, T2, and T2* are exponential decays
    C. The time constant T2* is always longer than the time constant T2 in practice
    D. Spin-spin relaxation is the decay of transverse magnetisation
    E. Resonance does not occur if the radiofrequency pulse is delivered at a different frequency to the Larmor frequency of the nucleus

---

After a radiofrequency pulse at the Larmor frequency has been applied and removed, relaxation processes occur resulting in a decrease in the amplitude of the net magnetic vector in the transverse plane. Thus the voltage measured by the receiver coil decreases. This is known as free induction decay.

Spin-lattice energy transfer: this reflects nuclei shifting their magnetic moments from high to low energy states with the energy exchanged to their surrounding environment. T1 recovery is a reflection of the efficiency of this exponential process (time taken for 63% of **longitudinal** magnetisation to recover). Fat is able to absorb energy quickly and T1 is short; water is inefficient at receiving energy from nuclei so T1 is longer.

Loss of precessional coherence: NMV decays in **transverse** plane by:

- **Spin-spin energy transfer**: interactions of the intrinsic magnetic fields of adjacent nuclei. This is described by T2 decay (time for 63% of transverse magnetisation to be lost due to dephasing). Fat is much better at this energy exchange than water (molecular motion matches Larmor frequency better) so T2 time is short.
- **Inhomogeneities of external magnetic field**: are inevitable in current magnets. As magnetic field strength is part of the Larmor equation, nuclei within inhomogeneities will precess at slightly different frequencies and diphase. This

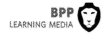

exponential process is known as T2* decay and precedes T2 decay 'proper'.

The TR controls how much of the longitudinal NMV in fat or water has recovered before the next RF pulse (thus how much differential T1 contrast is seen diminishes over time). The TE controls how much transverse magnetisation has been allowed to decay in fat and water when the signal is read (T2 contrast—exaggerated over time). Long TEs allow dephasing of the transverse components in fat and water, so demonstrating a contrast difference.

Proton density weighting seeks to diminish the effects of differences in T1 recovery and T2 decay within tissues, to produce an image whose contrast is predominantly due to differences in proton density (ie long TR and short TE).

---

13. A. **False** – T2 is the time taken for 63% of the transverse magnetisation to be lost
    B. **True** – these are exponential decay curves
    C. **False** – T2* is shorter than T2 in practice, as spin coherence is influenced by other factors (eg local magnetic field inhomogeneities). T2* denotes *observed* decay constant
    D. **True** – spin-spin relaxation is also termed T2 decay
    E. **True** – resonance will only occur at the Larmor frequency of the nucleus

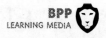

14. Regarding MRI
    A. The magnetic field requires homogeneity of 0.5 parts per million
    B. Resistive magnets are cooled using cryogenic fluids (eg liquid helium)
    C. SNR is reduced in direct proportion to a decrease in slice thickness
    D. An increase in the field of view can be used to overcome an aliasing artefact
    E. The signal-to-noise increases as the square of the number of excitations

Magnet field inhomogeneities are unavoidable in scanners, as electromagnet coils cannot be evenly spaced. Current-carrying (shim) coils are placed in the area of inhomogeneity to even this out. Inhomogeneities are measured in parts-per-million and homogeneity of below approximately 10 ppm is required for conventional imaging.

Resistive magnet field strength is dependent upon the current passing through its coils; the maximum field strength in a system of this type is less than 0.5 T due to excessive power requirements.

Signal-to-noise ratio is the ratio of useful MR signal to background noise. SNR is increased by increasing field strength; using phased coil arrays; long TR; short TE; large flip angles; increasing number of signal averages; reducing received bandwidth; and imaging proton-dense structures.

Aliasing (or phase-wrapping) occurs when tissue produces signal outside the FOV in the phase direction, and there is duplication of phase values for tissue inside and outside the FOV. Aliasing is reduced or eliminated by increasing the FOV to the boundaries of the coil; or by placing a spatial pre-saturation pulse over signal-producing areas; or by oversampling in the phase direction.

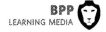

14. A. **False** – field homogeneity of 10 ppm is required for conventional MRI
     B. **False** – resistive magnets tend to be water-cooled
     C. **True** – thin slices are noisy
     D. **True** – aliasing occurs because the imaged object is larger than the chosen FOV
     E. **False** – SNR increases as the square root of the number of excitations

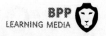

15.   Regarding spin echo pulse sequence
       A.   T1 recovery of fat is shorter than T1 recovery of
            water
       B.   T2 decay time of water is approximately 10 ms
       C.   Hydrogen in water loses transverse magnetisation
            slower than hydrogen in fat
       D.   T2 decay time of fat is approximately 80 ms
       E.   The strength of signal produced in a T1-weighted
            image is inversely proportional to the amount of
            transverse magnetisation produced after application
            of the RF pulse

T1 recovery is a reflection of the efficiency of the exponential process
(time taken for 63% of **longitudinal** magnetisation to recover) of
spin-lattice energy transfer. Fat is able to absorb energy quickly
and T1 is short; water is inefficient at receiving energy from nuclei
so T1 is longer.

T2 decay (time for 63% of **transverse** magnetisation to be lost due
to dephasing) is due to spin-spin energy transfer. Fat is much better
at this energy exchange than water (molecular motion matches
Larmor frequency better) so T2 time is short.

---

15.   A.   **True** – T1 recovery is shorter in fat which thus has
                      higher signal on T1 weighted CSE
       B.   **False** – T2 decay time of water is approximately 200
                       ms
       C.   **True** – hydrogen in fat recovers more rapidly along the
                      longitudinal axis than water, and loses transverse
                      magnetisation faster than water
       D.   **True** – T2 decay time of fat is approximately 80 ms
       E.   **False** – the signal in T1 weighted CSE is proportional
                       to the amount of transverse magnetisation
                       after RF pulse application (eg there is more
                       transverse magnetisation in fat than water, so
                       it is brighter)

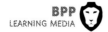

16. Regarding MRI design
    A. Resistive magnets can operate at field strengths of up to 0.5 T
    B. Clinical spectrometry requires a magnet with a field strength of between 0.2 and 0.4 Tesla
    C. Increasing the field of view decreases the signal-to-noise ratio
    D. SNR decreases as the data acquisition bandwidth decreases
    E. Nuclei with a nuclear spin value (I) of zero are suitable for MRI

Resistive magnet field strength uses the law of electromagnetic induction and is dependent upon the current passing through the magnet's coils. The maximum field strength in a system of this type is less than 0.5 T due to high power requirements.

Magnetic resonance spectroscopy provides a frequency spectrum of a tissue based on the molecular and chemical structures of that tissue (mostly using hydrogen, but advanced forms are able to evaluate other MR-active nuclei).

Signal-to-noise ratio is the ratio of useful MR signal to background noise. SNR is increased by increasing field strength, using phased coil arrays; long TR; short TE; large flip angles; increasing number of signal averages; reducing received bandwidth; and imaging proton-dense structures.

The nuclear spin value is always zero, a multiple of 0.5, or a whole number. Nuclei with a nuclear spin value of zero do not precess in a magnetic field.

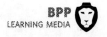

16. A. **True** – the maximum field strength of this system is less than 0.5 T
    B. **False** – spectrometry requires field strength of 1–2 Tesla
    C. **False** – increasing FOV increases voxel volume, and so contains more spins
    D. **False** – reducing the data acquisition bandwidth results in less noise being sampled relative to signal (but results in increased chemical shift artefact)
    E. **False** – nuclei with spin values other than zero are suitable for MRI

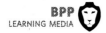

17.   Regarding the MRI scanner
       A.   Shim coils are used to perform phase encoding
       B.   Gradient fields are used to perform slice selection
       C.   There are four sets of gradient coils
       D.   The gradient, shim and RF coils lie between the
            magnet and the patient
       E.   Slice thickness can be altered by changing the
            bandwidth of the applied RF pulse

Gradients are coils of wire that alter the magnetic field of the magnet in a linear fashion when a current is passed through them. They are usually situated deep to the RF coils and change the magnetic field strength in a predictable fashion. By doing so, they change the precessional frequency (encoding the long axis) and phase (encoding the short axis) of magnetic moments of nuclei, and enable encoding of the MR signal in three dimensions.

The slice select gradient is switched on during the delivery of the RF excitation pulse (3.2 ms in the positive direction). The phase encoding gradient is switched on after the RF excitation pulse has been switched off (4 ms). The frequency encoding gradient is switched on during the echo (8 ms).

17.   A.   **False** – gradient coils are used for frequency and
                 phase encoding; shim coils smooth field
                 inhomogeneity
       B.   **True** – gradient fields are central to slice selection
       C.   **False** – there are three sets of coils that generate field
                 gradients in perpendicular directions
       D.   **True** – these coils lie within the inside diameter of the
                 magnet
       E.   **True** – slice thickness is also modified by altering the
                 steepness of the gradient field

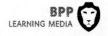

18. Regarding MRI contrast agents
    A. Gadolinium is a superparamagnetic agent
    B. Iron oxides result in signal loss in normal tissues on PD or heavily T2 weighted images
    C. Gadolinium cannot be excreted by the body in its pure form
    D. Gadolinium is contra-indicated in sickle cell anaemia
    E. Gadolinium is the contrast agent of choice in liver imaging

---

Gadolinium is a paramagnetic agent with seven unpaired electrons, and has properties which allow rapid exchange of water and minimise the space between itself and body water. The T1 relaxation times of the nearby water protons are reduced and results in increased signal on T1 weighted images (hence gadolinium is a T1 enhancement agent). Gadolinium cannot be excreted by the body and would cause adverse effects due to membrane binding. It is therefore bound with a chelate such as DTPA to enable safe excretion. Side-effects can include transient hyperbilirubinaemia and blood iron; rash; GI upset; headaches; nausea; vomiting and hypotension. Contraindications include haemolytic anaemia and pregnancy. Gadolinium is used extensively in CNS imaging as it passes through breakdowns in the BBB.

Iron oxides are used mainly in liver imaging where the normal liver is dark on T2 weighting and lesions are bright. Iron oxides shorten relaxation times of nearby hydrogen atoms and reduce the signal intensity in normal tissues. Superparamagnetic iron oxides are known as T2 enhancement agents and cause signal loss on PD- and T2- weighted images. Side-effects may include GI upset, moderate back, leg and groin pain, and in rare cases anaphylactoid reactions. It is contraindicated in patients with known allergies to iron and parenteral dextran.

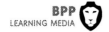

18.　A.　**False** – gadolinium is a paramagnetic agent
　　　B.　**True** – iron oxides result in T2 enhancement
　　　C.　**True** – gadolinium must be bound with a chelate for this reason
　　　D.　**True** – gadolinium is contraindicated in haemolytic disorders such as sickle cell anaemia
　　　E.　**False** – iron oxides are the agents of choice in liver disorder imaging

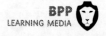

19. Regarding MRI
    A. Hydrogen and fluorine are MR active
    B. Chemical shift artefacts are decreased at higher magnetic field strengths
    C. Chemical shift artefacts are worse with larger fields of view
    D. Chemical shift artefacts can be reduced by increasing the receive band width
    E. Chemical shift artefacts are observed in the phase encoding direction

---

Protons and neutrons within a nucleus spin about their own axes in a random fashion (clockwise or anticlockwise); when there are an equal number of spinning nucleons they will tend to cancel one another out. A nucleus with an odd mass number will have net spin, and (given that protons have charge) net charge. A moving unbalanced charge induces a magnetic field, and this forms the basis of MR imaging.

Chemical shift artefact causes a signal void between fat and water interface, and results from the differences in molecular architecture of fat and water. This process causes slightly different precessional frequencies of hydrogen nuclei in either molecule.

Hydrogen in fat resonates at a lower frequency than water. This causes a frequency shift that increases with increasing field strength. The receive bandwidth controls chemical shift as well as influencing SNR, determining the range of frequencies mapped across each of pixels in the frequency axis of the FOV. Reducing receive bandwidth increases chemical artefact, since fewer frequencies are mapped across the same number of pixels. Chemical artefact is corrected by using lower field strengths or broadening the receive bandwidth. (One can also suppress water or fat signal using inversion sequences or pre-saturation).

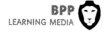

19. A. **True** – a nucleus with an odd mass number will be MR active
    B. **False** – chemical shift artefact is increased with higher magnetic field strengths
    C. **True** – chemical shift artefact is more pronounced when using larger fields of view
    D. **True** – chemical shift artefact can be reduced by using an increased receive bandwidth
    E. **False** – chemical shift artefacts are observed only in the frequency encoding axis

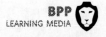

20. Regarding MRI safety
 A. A Faraday cage surrounds the MR scanner to shield it from external electromagnetic fields
 B. The level of restriction around a clinical MR area for members of the public is around 0.01 Tesla
 C. Staff are not permitted to be in the scan room during the sequence
 D. Abdominal surgical clips are generally safe for MR
 E. Manual quenching should be performed on a regular basis as part of a safety programme

---

Due to the safety considerations of a 'permanent' magnetic field it is prudent and mandatory for all persons entering the controlled areas to satisfy a safety screening process.

As the resonance frequency of protons is very close to that of the radio waves used in radio broadcasting and the FM band, the MR device is placed in a Faraday cage to insulate it from external RF signals which could alter the signal. The copper Faraday cage completely encases the MR scanner.

There are two levels of safety zones around the installation. The 'exclusion zone' is defined by the 5 Gauss line (good practice suggests this line actually is located within the exclusion zone). This may be expressed as 0.0005 T (1 Tesla ≡ 20,000 Gauss). The 'security' zone is where the potential for projectile injuries occurs (usually the scan room).

Staff are not usually exposed to the static magnet field when in the control room, however occasions may require them to be present in the scan room (eg for monitoring or dynamic investigations).

Quenching is the process whereby the cryobath is vented; the superconducting coils lose their low temperature and become resistive (and therefore the magnetic field is lost). Manual quenching is instigated in extreme emergencies (such as a ferromagnetic object pinning an individual to the magnet). It has significant potential to

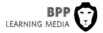

severely and irreversibly damage the coils. The cryogenic material should undergo automatic venting in this scenario.

---

20.   A.   **True** – this usually copper shielding is vital to prevent external radiofrequencies compromising the accuracy of signals received

    B.   **False** – the exclusion zone is defined by the 5 Gauss line, which equates to 0.0005 T

    C.   **False** – this may be required for patient monitoring, reassurance or intervention

    D.   **True** – abdominal surgical clips are generally well anchored and safe, but may result in artefact

    E.   **False** – manual quenching should only be used in emergency situations and results in severe damage to the superconducting coils

Chapter 15
Ultrasound

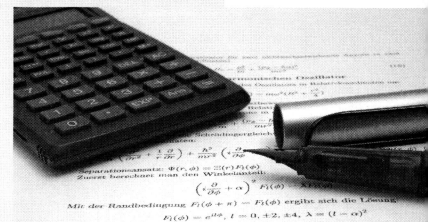

Ultrasound

Please answer all questions true or false. There is no negative marking.

> 1. Ultrasound has the following typical properties
>   A. It is a transverse wave
>   B. The unit of frequency Hertz (Hz) equals 10^3 cycles per second
>   C. The frequency of individual transducers is fixed
>   D. The intensity of US is under the operator's control
>   E. The transmitter and receiver are the same

Ultrasound is simply sound waves, like audible sound. Although some physical properties are different as a result of the change in frequency, the basic principles are the same.

Sound consists of waves of compression and decompression of the transmitting medium (eg air or water), travelling at a fixed velocity. Sound is an example of a longitudinal wave oscillating back and forth in the direction the sound wave travels, thus consisting of successive zones of compression and rarefaction. Transverse waves are oscillations in the transverse direction of the propagation, eg electromagnetic radiation.

The hertz (Hz) is the (SI) unit of frequency. It is defined as the number of cycles per second. 1 Hz is equal to one cycle per second.

1. A. **False** – it is a longitudinal wave
    B. **False** – 1 Hz equals 1 cycle per second
    C. **True** – ultrasound transducers have a fixed frequency
    D. **True** – there is a control on the ultrasound machine
    E. **True** – the probe and its piezoelectric crystal act as the transducer and the receiver

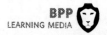

2.   Regarding sound
A.   Audible frequencies are in the range of 1–12 MHz
B.   Ultrasound can bend around corners
C. $c = \lambda f$
D.   It travels with the same velocity in air as it does in water
E.   Sound waves consist of successive zones of compression and rarefaction

---

Diagnostic ultrasound is in the range of 1–12 MHz.

Audible sound can be heard around a corner. The higher frequencies used in ultrasound result is sound waves travelling in straighter lines, thus it is not able to bend around corners. At higher frequencies the ultrasound behaves more like electromagnetic radiation.

The wavelength λ is inversely related to the frequency f by the sound velocity c, where:

$$c = \lambda f$$

meaning that the velocity equals the wavelength times the number of oscillations per second, and thus:

$$\lambda = c/f$$

The velocity of sound in a given medium is constant and dependent upon the compressibility and density of the medium. The greater the density and the compressibility of a medium, the lower is the velocity of the ultrasound wave.

---

2.   A.   **False** – audible sound frequencies are below 15,000 to 20,000 Hz
B.   **False** – ultrasound cannot travel around corners
C.   **True** – velocity = wavelength times frequency
D.   **False** – US travels in air at 330 m/s and in water at 1540 m/s
E.   **True** – sound waves consist of successive zones of compression and rarefaction

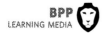

> 3. Concerning the piezoelectric effect
>   A. It is the ability of some materials to generate an electrical response to an applied mechanical stress
>   B. It is the ability of some materials to generate a mechanical stress following an applied electrical response
>   C. It is affected by temperature
>   D. It is used in the production and detection of sound
>   E. The standard piezoelectric material for medical imaging processes has been lead zirconate titanate (PZT)

Piezolectric elements have the ability to convert an applied voltage into sound waves, and sound waves into a voltage. In clinical practice, microcrystalline lead zirconate titanate or plastic polyvinylidine difluoride are used. They are coated with a thin layer of silver for electrical conducting.

The Curie temperature is used to describe the temperature above which the material loses its spontaneous piezoelectric characteristics.

---

3. A. **True** – piezolectric elements have the ability to convert electric current into mechanical movement and vice versa
   B. **True** – see above
   C. **True** – piezoelectric effect is lost above the Curie temperature
   D. **True** – used in the production and detection of sound
   E. **True** – the standard piezoelectric material for medical imaging processes has been lead zirconate titanate (PZT)

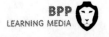

4.	In ultrasound
	A.	The velocity of transmission in the body is dependent on the US frequency
	B.	The lower the density of a medium, the higher the velocity of the ultrasound wave
	C.	In order to see the reflective surface it is desirable that the incident beam strikes tissue surfaces as nearly as possible to right angles
	D.	The reflective surface will be seen if the densities of the media on each side of the boundary are different
	E.	In order to see the reflective surface, the reflective surface must be stationary

The velocity of ultrasound is dependent on tissue characteristics such as density and compressibility. It does not change with frequency. The greater the density and the compressibility of a medium, the lower the velocity of the ultrasound wave.

In order to see reflective surfaces, there must be a difference in acoustic impedance between tissues. Acoustic impedance is *density x speed* of sound. If a reflective surface is struck at right angles, the maximum number of echoes will be returned to the probe. At a smaller angle, some of the returning echoes will not reach the probe and less energy will return to the transducer.

4.	A.	**False** – velocity does not change with frequency
	B.	**True** – the greater the density, the lower the velocity of the ultrasound wave
	C.	**True** – at right angles the largest amount of the beam will return to the transducer
	D.	**True** – in order to see the reflective surface it is actually acoustic impedance that must change
	E.	**False** – heart valve, vessel walls etc. are not stationary but can still be seen

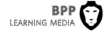

5. Regarding the pulse-echo principle
   A. More information about the location and size of the reflector can be obtained if the beam is narrow
   B. The speed of sound in most soft tissues is similar
   C. The strength of the echoes decreases with depth
   D. If you hear an echo in a mountain range 6 seconds after you have created a scream, the reflecting mountain is 1980 m away (given sound travels at 330 m/s in air)
   E. TGC can be manually altered

All ultrasound is performed on the pulse-echo principle. A pulse is sent out that partially reflects as it encounters structures in the body. Then the echoes from the reflected pulse are received. The times at which the echoes are received are representative of the distance to those objects. This is described by the formula below.

$$R = ct/2$$

(where R = distance, c = speed of sound in tissue, and t = time.)

The velocity of ultrasound in soft tissue is assumed to be relatively constant at 1540 m/s. This aids in calculating distances.

Echo amplitudes received at the transducer gradually reduce as depth increases. This is because some of the signal is lost (attenuated) on the way. The machine is therefore equipped with a control which allows the operator to adjust the amount of gain (amplification) which is applied to echoes from different depths. This is called Time Gain Compensation (TGC), and is an important control for the operator to identify and master.

5. A. **True** – a narrow beam allows for better resolution
   B. **True** – the speed of sound in most soft tissues is = 1340 m/s
   C. **True** – increasing depth results in increased attenuation, thus returning echoes are less
   D. **False** – the reflecting mountain is 990 m away
   E. **True** – TGC can be manually altered

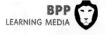

> 6. Regarding the structure of an ultrasound transducer
>   A. The backing layer material has similar acoustic impedance to the transducer
>   B. The resonant frequency is related to the thickness of the piezoelectric disk
>   C. The sound wave produced in pulse echo undergoes dampening and ringing
>   D. Heavy dampening results in a long time constant
>   E. Light dampening relates to a high Q

An ultrasound transducer is made of (from front to back): a thin plastic slip, a piezoelectric disc and a backing block. A voltage is applied to the back of the piezoelectric disc and the front face is connected to an earthed metal case.

The voltage applied to the piezoelectric disc results in it "ringing" at its resonant frequency. The ultrasound wave travels in all directions from the disc. The backing layer is matched to the piezoelectric disc in order to dampen this "ringing" and provide a short pulse. A short pulse is important for good axial resolution.

The thin front plastic slip has an acoustic impedance somewhere in between that of the piezoelectric disc and the examined tissue. This aids the transference of the ultrasound waves to the tissue.

The fundamental resonant frequency is achieved when thickness of the piezoelectric disc $= \lambda/2$.

6. A. **True** – so the wave is transmitted rather then reflected
    B. **True** – and the material used
    C. **True** – the sound wave produced in pulse echo undergoes dampening and ringing
    D. **False** – heavy dampening results in a short time constant
    E. **True** – a transducer that is lightly damp has a high Q

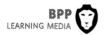

7. Regarding ultrasound
    A. In pulsed mode, a range of sound waves with different frequencies are emitted
    B. A short pulse will have a wider bandwidth than a long pulse
    C. Mechanical co-efficient (Q) is the ratio of mean frequency to bandwidth
    D. High Q probes produce and receive only one pure note
    E. High Q probes are good for continuous wave ultrasound

Once the transducer is pulsed a sound wave is produced. The amplitude of the sound wave decays exponentially with time. This is known as dampening. Vibrations that continue for some time are known as ringing. Heavy dampening results in a short time constant or ring-down time. This is known as a low Q. Light dampening results in a long time constant or ring-down time, known as a high Q. A transducer with a high Q produces a longer constant and a higher output of sound.

Continuous mode sound of a single frequency is emitted. In pulsed mode a spectrum of sound waves of different frequencies are emitted. The full width at half maximum height of the total intensity (FWHM) is known as the bandwidth.

Short pulses have wider bandwidth than long pulses. The ratio of the mean frequency to the bandwidth denotes the mechanical co-efficient Q. The table below depicts what ultrasound characteristics are useful for which modality.

Mechanical co-efficient	Bandwidth	Ultrasound type
High Q	Narrower bandwidth	Continuous wave ultrasound
Low Q	Wider bandwidth	Pulsed ultrasound

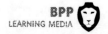

7. A. **True** – a continuous spectrum with sounds of different frequencies is emitted
    B. **True** – a short pulse will have a wider bandwidth than a long pulse
    C. **True** – mechanical co-efficient (Q) is the ratio of mean frequency to bandwidth
    D. **True** – this is true
    E. **False** – a high Q probe is good for continuous wave ultrasound

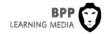

8. The following are true
   A. The ultrasound beam is made up of (nearly) parallel sound waves throughout
   B. Fresnel zone is the near field
   C. The higher the frequency, the longer the near field
   D. The angle of divergence is proportional to the wavelength
   E. A high frequency transducer will have an increased attenuation

The ultrasound beam is made up of a near (Fresnel) zone consisting of nearly parallel waves and a far (Fraunhofer) zone consisting of divergent ultrasound waves.

The length of the near zone is calculated by:

$$D^2 / 4\lambda = fD^2$$

The angle of divergence of the far zone is calculated by:

$$\lambda/D = fD$$

Thus a high frequency ultrasound beam will have a longer area of nearly parallel waves, which is useful for imaging. However, a higher frequency beam will have less penetration as a result of increased attenuation.

8. A. **False** – the near part of the ultrasound beam is made up of (nearly) parallel sound waves
   B. **True** – Frauenhofer zone is known as the far field
   C. **True** – the higher the frequency, the longer the near field
   D. **False** – the angle of divergence is inversely proportional to the wavelength
   E. **True** – higher frequency results in increased attenuation

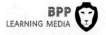

9. In ultrasound imaging
    A. dB is the unit of acoustic impedance
    B. Acoustic impedance is the product of density and frequency
    C. At the interface between tissues of similar acoustic impedance, a small proportion of the beam is reflected
    D. Absorption of ultrasound in tissues results in heat production
    E. The thickness of the piezoelectric crystals should be equal to the wavelength of the US to be produced

Acoustic impedance is the product of density of the material and the velocity of sound. The differences in acoustic impedance of two materials at a boundary dictate the amount of reflection or transmission that occurs at the junction between the two materials. The angle of incidence is also important.

Sound attenuation through a material increases with an exponential relationship to distance travelled within the material. The unit of attenuation is the decibel.

9. A. **False** – dB is the unit of attenuation
    B. **False** – acoustic impedance is the product of density and speed
    C. **True** – a smaller proportion of the beam is reflected at interface of similar acoustic impedance
    D. **True** – absorption of ultrasound in tissues results in heat production
    E. **False** – resonant frequency occurs at half a wavelength thickness

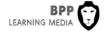

> 10. Regarding A-mode imaging
>   A. It is no longer applied alone in modern-day ultrasound
>   B. It is the simplest form of ultrasound imaging
>   C. Time gain compensation is an electronic adjustment of the received pulse
>   D. Principles differ from modern-day ultrasound
>   E. It is a single US pulse, therefore it has poor lateral resolution

In A-mode imaging is the simplest form of imaging, standing for amplitude modulation. In this, a cathode-ray tube (CRT) is used to display a graph that has one axis representing the time required for the return of the echo, and the other corresponding to the strength of the echo. It has largely been superseded by B-mode ultrasound, but is still used for imaging the eye.

The pulse weakens the further it travels in the body, and so pulses received after some time undergo electronic amplification in order to compensate for this. This is known as time gain compensation (TGC). As it is a single beam, it will have no lateral resolution.

10. A. **False** – it is still used
    B. **True** – it is the original and simplest form
    C. **True** – TGC is an electronic adjustment
    D. **False** – modern-day ultrasound works on the same basic principles
    E. **True** – a minimum of two pulses are required for lateral resolution

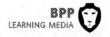

11. Regarding B-mode imaging
    A. 'B' stands for boldness
    B. It results in a picture formed of several echoes
    C. It has better lateral resolution than A-mode
    D. Multiple focal zones impact on real-time imaging
    E. Mechanical scanners are employed in B-mode scanning

B-mode stands for brightness mode sonography. In B-mode ultrasound, a linear array of transducers simultaneously scans a plane through the body that can be viewed as a two-dimensional image on screen.

A two-dimensional image is built up by firing a beam vertically, waiting for the return echoes; maintaining the information; and then firing a new beam from a neighbouring transducer along a neighbouring line in a sequence of B-mode lines.

Real-time imaging describes an image that is formed and renewed in a time shorter than that required for appreciable change in that structure. For this, a frame rate of 25 fps is required. Each frame is made up of several lines of acoustic information, incorporating the delay in sending and receiving the information. The natural compromise comes between amount of information and frame rate.

Multiple focal zones infer an increase in the amount of information. Thus the frame rate slows and real-time imaging is compromised.

Both mechanical and electronic sector scanners can be used in B-mode imaging.

11. A. **False** – 'B' stands for brightness mode
    B. **True** – the amplitude of echoes is allocated a grey-scale setting
    C. **True** – has better lateral resolution than A-mode
    D. **True** – these slow down scanning, but offer greater detail
    E. **True** – as well as electronic scanners

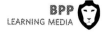

> 12. In a linear phased array
>   A. The footprint refers to the width of the probe
>   B. Sequential vertical beams are fired
>   C. The field of view is smaller than the footprint of the probe
>   D. There is a small near field
>   E. There is a large sector size

In a linear array of ultrasound crystals, the electronic phased array shoots parallel beams in sequence, creating a field that is as wide as the probe length (footprint).

A curvilinear array has a curved surface, creating a depth in the field that is wider than the footprint of the probe, making it possible to create a smaller footprint for easier access through small windows. This will result in a wider field but at the cost of reduced lateral resolution as the scan lines diverge.

The linear array gives a large probe surface (footprint) and near field, and a narrow sector. A curvilinear array will also give a large footprint and near field, but with a wide sector.

12. A. **True** – the footprint refers to the width of the probe
    B. **True** – sequential vertical beams are fired
    C. **False** – the field of view is as wide as the footprint
    D. **False** – there is a large near field
    E. **False** – there is a narrow sector size

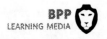

13. Regarding resolution in ultrasound
    A. Lateral resolution depends upon pulse length
    B. Lateral resolution depends upon frequency
    C. Lateral resolution depends upon beam width
    D. Axial resolution depends upon beam width
    E. Axial resolution depends upon frequency

Lateral resolution is the ability to separate two structures alongside each other at a particular scan depth. It depends upon frequency, machine focus setting and beam width.

Axial resolution is the ability to separate two structures that lie in the same scan line. It depends upon pulse length and frequency.

13. A. **False** – lateral resolution is independent of pulse length
    B. **True** – lateral resolution depends upon frequency
    C. **True** – lateral resolution depends upon beam width
    D. **False** – axial resolution is independent of beam width
    E. **True** – axial resolution depends upon frequency

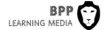

> 14. Phase-arrayed ultrasound can vary
>   A. Direction of beam
>   B. Focal length
>   C. Axial resolution
>   D. Lateral resolution
>   E. Pulse repetition frequency

All elements of an electronic sector scanner can be energised at the same time to create a beam that travels in the forward direction. Alternatively, if the elements are energised sequentially they will result in the beam swinging in one direction. If the order of energisation is reversed, the beam will swing in the other direction. This is known as steered or phased array.

Sequential firing of the individual elements can control the direction of the beam and the focal length. Lateral resolution depends on beam width which is affected by focusing.

14. A. **True** – phase-arrayed ultrasound can vary direction of beam
    B. **True** – phase-arrayed ultrasound can vary focal length
    C. **True** – phase-arrayed ultrasound can vary axial resolution
    D. **True** – phase-arrayed ultrasound can vary lateral resolution
    E. **True** – phase-arrayed ultrasound can vary pulse repetition frequency

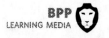

15. Regarding the safety of ultrasound
    A. The detrimental effects of US are thought to arise solely from its thermal effects
    B. It is particularly important in obstetric examination
    C. Exposure time is an irrelevant factor in relation to temperature rise
    D. The thermal index is referred to in the BMUS guidelines
    E. There is evidence of harmful effects at current exposure levels

---

Whilst ultrasound is a safe imaging modality not utilising electromagnetic radiation, it is still important to be aware of its potential detrimental effects. These can vary from local heating, cavitations, changes in cell permeability and mechanical damage to cell membranes.

Agreed safety guidelines recommend that the time-averaged intensity should not exceed 100 mW/cm2; and that the total sound energy (intensity x scan time) should not be in excess of 50 J/cm2.

The thermal index is the ratio of the power emitted to that required to increase temperature by one degree Centigrade. It indicates the degree of tissue heating due to absorption of ultrasound energy.

---

15. A. **False** – mechanical effects are also important
    B. **True** – theoretically the foetus is more sensitive to thermal and mechanical effects
    C. **False** – exposure time is relevant
    D. **True** – the thermal index is the basis of the BMUS guidelines
    E. **False** – there is no evidence of harmful effects at current operative levels

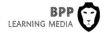

16. Regarding artefacts in ultrasound
    A. Result from assumptions about the behaviour of the sound wave
    B. Speckling is a result of interference between sound waves reflected from numerous small structures
    C. Acoustic shadowing occurs when sound passes through fluid-filled structures
    D. Reverberation and ring-down artefact are the same entity
    E. Acoustic enhancement occurs posterior to gas-containing structures

Ultrasound image formation assumes certain behaviour characteristics of ultrasound. It presumes that all ultrasound waves travel in straight lines at the same velocity, and behave in the same way when they come across different structures at any depth.

Speckling is the result of interference between sound waves reflected from numerous small structures. The structures themselves are too small to be seen, but the interaction of their echoes can result in a typical picture with a characteristic echo texture for a particular organ.

Acoustic shadowing: bowel gas, lung bone and stones are all highly attenuating structures. On ultrasound these will give posterior anechoic strips called shadows.

Acoustic enhancement: weakly attenuating structures such as cysts will have a posterior hyperechoic stripe known as enhancement.

---

16. A. **True** – result from assumptions about the behaviour of the sound wave
    B. **True** – speckling is a result of interference between sound waves reflected from numerous small structures
    C. **False** – acoustic enhancement occurs when sound passes through fluid filled structures
    D. **False** – they are not the same entity
    E. **False** – acoustic shadowing occurs posterior to gas containing structures

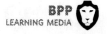

17. Regarding artefacts in ultrasound
   A. Acoustic enhancement is a result of sound travelling at different speeds through different structures
   B. Acoustic shadowing is a result of strongly attenuating structures reducing the intensity of echoes received from behind
   C. Edge-shadowing artefact is a result of attenuation and refraction at the edge of a structure
   D. Ring-down artefact and comet–tail artefact are the same entity
   E. Double reflections are common at the diaphragm

Ring–down: a resonating gas bubble continuously emits ultrasound, resulting in a track often appearing like a comet-tail.

Double reflection: highly reflective structures such as the diaphragm can give the appearance that the liver is duplicated in the thorax.

17. A. **False** – acoustic enhancement is a result of increased intensity of echoes arising posterior to a fluid-filled structure. This is because the anterior (poorly attenuating) structure has allowed a greater intensity of ultrasound through, and therefore a greater intensity of ultrasound is reflected back
   B. **True** – acoustic shadowing is a result of strongly attenuating structures reducing the intensity of echoes received from behind
   C. **True** – edge-shadowing artefact is a result of attenuation and refraction at the edge of a structure
   D. **True** – ring-down artefact and comet–tail artefact are the same entity
   E. **True** – double reflections are common at the diaphragm

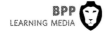

18. Regarding quality assurance in ultrasound
    A. A sheet phantom is used
    B. A calorimeter measures the heating effect, and hence the power output
    C. A perspex block is used as no adjustments need to be made with regard to the speed of sound
    D. Dynamic range and A-scan calliper measurements require tissue-mimicking phantoms
    E. Grey-scale performance and resolution can be checked on the same test rig

Quality assurance in ultrasound requires numerous tools. The table below provides a suitable summary.

Test	Tool
Resolution	Test rig composed of parallel wires immersed in a water bath contained in a perspex box
Sensitivity, dynamic range and accuracy of the A-scan calliper	Perspex box with parallel vertical rods
Grey-scale performance and Doppler function	Tissue-equivalent phantoms
Power output	A force balance can 'weigh' pressure A calorimeter can be used to measure heating

18. A. **False** – a sheet phantom is used in PET
    B. **True** – this is one method
    C. **False** – sound travels faster in perspex and corrections will be made for this
    D. **False** – these can be performed on a perspex block
    E. **False** – grey-scale performance requires a tissue-equivalent phantom

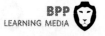

19. Regarding the Doppler effect
    A. It produces a change in the velocity of sound reflected off a moving object
    B. The frequency of the reflected ultrasound waves decreases if the interface is moving towards the transducer
    C. It requires the US beam to be near-parallel to the direction of movement to give the largest change in frequency
    D. It produces a change in frequency which is inversely proportional to the velocity of sound in the medium
    E. It requires a higher frequency than would be used for imaging

---

The Doppler effect describes the change in wavelength and frequency that occurs in an ultrasound wave when it encounters a moving source. If the source is moving towards the receiver, the reflected wave will have an increase in frequency; and if it is moving away there will be a decrease in frequency.

The change in frequency known as the Doppler shift is equal to:

$$2VF \cos \theta / C$$

where:
θ = the angle of insonation (note $\cos 90 = 0$, therefore there is no Doppler shift when the probe is perpendicular to the vessel; and being parallel to the vessel direction gives largest frequency shift as $\cos 0 = 1$)
F = frequency of the beam
C = velocity of sound in tissue
V = velocity of the interface

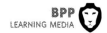

19.   A.   **False** – the velocity of sound is always constant within a given medium
      B.   **False** – it increases
      C.   **True** – this gives the largest frequency shift
      D.   **True** – the Doppler effect produces a change in frequency which is inversely proportional to the velocity of sound in the medium
      E.   **False** – no change in frequency is required

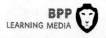

> 20. Regarding the Doppler effect
>   A. There is a maximum velocity which can be detected
>   B. The maximum Doppler shift frequency detected is half the pulse repetition frequency
>   C. Aliasing is a result of Doppler shift frequency exceeding half of the pulse repetition frequency
>   D. The pulsatility index is a qualitative measurement deduced from the Doppler signal
>   E. The resistance index is a quantitative measurement deduced from the Doppler signal

The Nyqvist limit states that the maximum Doppler effect detectable = PRF/2, where PRF is the number of ultrasound pulses produced per second.

Aliasing arises when Doppler shift frequency exceeds half of the PRF. This can be overcome by increasing PR if possible, changing the angle of scanning, or by reducing the scanning frequency and thus reducing the Doppler shift frequency.

Large changes in flow waveform shape are obvious; a quantitative measurement is useful in clinical practice. The resistance (or resistive) index RI, and pulsatility index PI, are based on measurements of the outline of the sonogram.

RI is calculated as:

Peak systolic frequency – end diastolic frequency/peak systolic frequency

PI is calculated as:

Peak systolic frequency – minimum frequency/time averaged maximum frequency

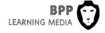

20. A. **False** – only with pulsed ultrasound
     B. **True** – maximum Doppler shift frequency detected is half the pulse repetition frequency
     C. **True** – aliasing arises when doppler shift frequency exceeds half of the PRF
     D. **False** – both are quantitative measurements
     E. **True** – see above

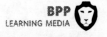

References

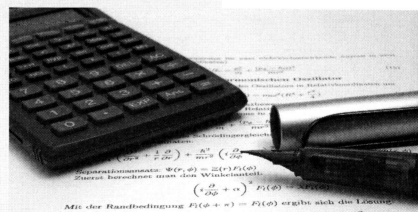

References

Allisy-Roberts P and Wiliams J (2008) *Farr's Physics for Medical Imaging*. 2nd edition. Philadelphia: Saunders Elsevier.

Dendy PP and Heaton B (1999) *Physics for Diagnostic Radiology*. 2nd edition. Abingdon: Taylor and Francis.

Health and Safety Commission (2000) *Work with Ionising Radiation L121 (Ionising Radiations Regulations 1999, Approved Code of Practice and Guidance)*. London: Health and Safety Executive.

Huda W and Slone R (2003) *Review of Radiologic Physics*. 2nd edition. Philadelphia: Lippincott Williams and Wilkins.

Powsner RA and Powsner ER (2006) *Essential Nuclear Medicine Physics*. 2nd edition. Oxford: Blackwell Publishing.

Tolan D, Hyland R, Taylor C and Cowen A (2004) *FRCR Part 1: MCQs and Mock Examinations*. London: Royal Society of Medicine Press.

Weissleder R, *et al.* (2006) *Primer of Diagnostic Imaging*. 4th edition. Philadelphia: Mosby.

Westbrook C, Roth CK and Talbot J (2005) *MRI in Practice*. 3rd edition. Oxford: Wiley-Blackwell.

Westbrook C (2002) *MRI at a Glance*. Oxford: Wiley-Blackwell.

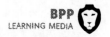

More titles in the Progressing your Medical Career Series

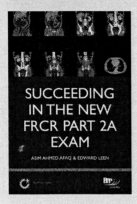

SUCCEEDING IN THE NEW FRCR PART 2A EXAM

ASIM AHMED AFAQ & EDWARD LEEN

£24.99
November 2011
Paperback
978-1-445379-52-4

Do you want to pass the FRCR Part 2a Exam first time and with a high score? Are you looking for practice SBAs with detailed answer explanations?

Succeeding in the FRCR Part 2a Exam is an essential part of completing radiology training. This comprehensive revision guide contains practice SBAs together with detailed answer explanations covering the six modules of the syllabus. Written by doctors who have successfully passed the FRCR Part 2a Exam together with a Professor of Radiology Teaching, the questions have been carefully created to simulate the style of the new format.

This clear and time-saving FRCR Part 2a SBA practice guide:

- Comprises over 300 SBA practice questions designed to provide optimal preparation for FRCR 2a candidates

- Addresses a wide range of topics within each of the 6 modules to help reinforce knowledge and uncover areas where further reading is needed

- References from which the questions were created are detailed, many of which are recent articles in major Radiology journals together with Radiology textbooks

This engaging and easy to use guide will enable you to gain valuable practice in preparation of FRCR Part 2a, and is an essential revision book for anyone serious about excelling in this exam.

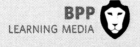

More titles in the Progressing your Medical Career Series

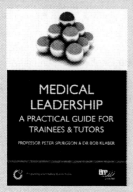

MEDICAL LEADERSHIP
A PRACTICAL GUIDE FOR TRAINEES & TUTORS

PROFESSOR PETER SPURGEON & DR BOB KLABER

£19.99

November 2011

Paperback

978-1-445379-57-9

Are you a doctor or medical student who wishes to acquire and develop your leadership and management skills? Do you recognise the role and influence of strong leadership and management in modern medicine?

Clinical leadership is something in which all doctors should have an important role in terms of driving forward high quality care for their patients. In this up-to-date guide Peter Spurgeon and Robert Klaber take you through the latest leadership and management thinking, and how this links in with the Medical Leadership Competency Framework. As well as influencing undergraduate curricula and some of the concepts underpinning revalidation, this framework forms the basis of the leadership component of the curricula for all medical specialties, so a practical knowledge of it is essential for all doctors in training.

Using case studies and practical exercises to provide a strong work-based emphasis, this practical guide will enable you to build on your existing experiences to develop your leadership and management skills, and to develop strategies and approaches to improving care for your patients.

This book addresses:

- Why strong leadership and management are crucial to delivering high quality care

- The theory and evidence behind the Medical Leadership Competency Framework

- The practical aspects of leadership learning in a wide range of clinical environments (eg handover, EM, ward etc)

- How Consultants and trainers can best facilitate leadership learning for their trainees and students within the clinical work-place

Whether you are a medical student just starting out on your career, or an established doctor wishing to develop yourself as a clinical leader, this practical, easy-to-use guide will give you the techniques and knowledge you require to excel.

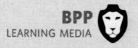

BPP
LEARNING MEDIA

www.bpp.com/health

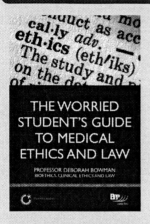
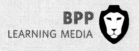

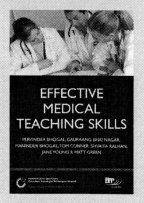
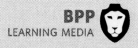

More titles in the Progressing your Medical Career Series

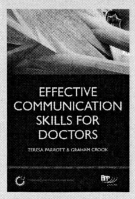

EFFECTIVE
COMMUNICATION
SKILLS FOR
DOCTORS

TERESA PARROTT & GRAHAM CROOK

£19.99

September 2011

Paperback

978-1-445379-56-2

Would you like to know how to improve your communication skills? Are you looking for a clearly written book which explores all aspects of effective medical communication?

There is an urgent need to improve doctors' communication skills. Research has shown that poor communication can contribute to patient dissatisfaction, lack of compliance and increased medico-legal problems. Improved communication skills will impact positively on all of these areas.

The last fifteen years have seen unprecedented changes in medicine and the role of doctors. Effective communication skills are vital to these new roles. But communication is not just related to personality. Skills can be learned which can make your communication more effective, and help you to improve your relationships with patients, their families and fellow doctors.

This book shows how to learn those skills and outlines why we all need to communicate more effectively. Healthcare is increasingly a partnership. Change is happening at all levels, from government directives to patient expectations. Communication is a bridge between the wisdom of the past and the vision of the future.

Readers of this book can also gain free access to an online module which upon successful completion can download a certificate for their portfolio of learning/ Revalidation/CPD records.

This easy-to-read guide will help medical students and doctors at all stages of their careers improve their communication within a hospital environment.

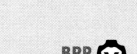
BPP
LEARNING MEDIA

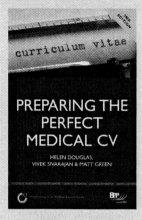
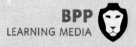

More titles in the Essential Clinical Handbook Series

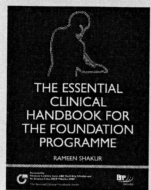

THE ESSENTIAL CLINICAL HANDBOOK FOR THE FOUNDATION PROGRAMME

RAMEEN SHAKUR

£24.99

October 2011

Paperback

978-1-445381-63-3

Unsure of what clinical competencies you must gain to successfully complete the Foundation Programme? Unclear on how to ensure your ePortfolio is complete to enable your progression to ST training?

This up-to-date clinical handbook is aimed at current foundation doctors and clinical medical students and provides a comprehensive companion to help you in the day-to-day management of patients on the ward. Together with this it is the first handbook to also outline clearly how to gain the core clinical competencies required for successful completion of the Foundation Programme. Written by doctors for doctors this comprehensive handbook explains how to successfully manage all of the common cases you will face during the Foundation Programme and:

- Introduces the Foundation Programme and what is expected of a new doctor especially with the introduction of Modernising Medical Careers

- Illustrates clearly the best way to manage, step-by-step, over 150 commonly encountered clinical diseases, including NICE guidelines to ensure a gold standard of clinical care is achieved.

- Describes how to successfully gain the core clinical competencies within Medicine and Surgery including an extensive list of differentials and conditions explained

- Explores the various radiology images you will encounter and how to interpret them

- Tells you how to succeed in the assessment methods used including DOP's, Mini-CEX's and CBD's.

- Has step by step diagrammatic guide to doing common clinical procedures competently and safely.

- Outlines how to ensure your ePortfolio is maintained properly to ensure successful completion of the Foundation Programme.

- Provides tips and advice on how to start preparing now to ensure you are fully prepared and have the competitive edge for your CMT/ST application.

The introduction of the e-Portfolio as part of the Foundation Programme has paved the way for foundation doctors to take charge of their own learning and portfolio. Through following the expert guidance laid down in this handbook you will give yourself the best possible chance of progressing successfully through to CMT/ST training.

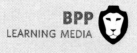

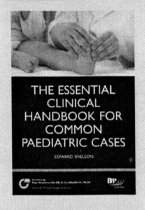
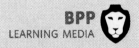